MW01101652

DASH Diet

The Complete Guide to Lose Weight, Lower Blood Pressure, and Stop Hypertension Fast With 60 Delicious and Easy DASH Diet Recipes

By

Mark Evans

The information in the following pages is broadly considered to be a truthful and accurate account of facts, and as such any inattention, use or misuse of the information in question by the reader will render any resulting actions solely under their purview. There are no scenarios in which the publisher or the original author of this work can be in any fashion deemed liable for any hardship or damages that may befall them after undertaking information described herein.

Additionally, the information found on the following pages is intended for informational purposes only and should thus be considered, universal. As befitting its nature, the information presented is without assurance regarding its continued validity or interim quality. Trademarks that mentioned are done without written consent and can in no way be considered an endorsement from the trademark holder.

Table of Contents

Part I

Part II

Part I

DASH Diet

Top 60 Delicious and Easy DASH Diet Recipes to Lose Weight, Lower Blood Pressure and Stop Hypertension Fast

CHAPTER 1

Brief Introduction to DASH Diet

The word "DASH" in DASH diet stands for **D**ietary **A**pproaches to **S**top **H**ypertension. As you can derive from its acronym, the DASH diet is a lifelong approach to instilling a healthy food lifestyle that can prevent or treat hypertension (high blood pressure). This diet aims to lower blood pressure by reducing sodium and adding more magnesium, calcium, and potassium into your diet. It also entails eating food that has high nutritional value.

In as early as two weeks, you will be able to reduce your blood pressure by following the DASH diet. By sticking to the plan, you can reduce 8 to 14 points from your systolic blood pressure which can make a significant difference to avoid both short- and long-term health risks.

Aside from reducing risk for hypertension, following the DASH diet can also prevent diabetes, stroke, heart disease, cancer, and osteoporosis.

Types of DASH Diet

The standard DASH diet encourages regular intake of low-fat dairy products, fruits, vegetables and allows moderate intake of nuts, poultry, fish, and whole grains. But, aside from the standard, there is also a lower sodium variation of the diet depending on your health needs.

The **standard DASH diet** allows for 2,300mg of sodium per day while the **lower sodium DASH diet** limits your intake to 1,500mg of sodium per day. The standard DASH diet follows the recommended daily allowance for sodium intake which is less than 2,300mg per day. While the lower sodium version acts as an upper limit and is only recommended if endorsed by your physician.

What to Eat

Whether you are on the standard or lower sodium version of DASH diet, expect to include a lot of low-fat dairy products, vegetables, fruits, and whole grains to your diet. Adding small amounts of seeds and nuts, legumes, poultry, and fish a few times per week is also encouraged.

A typical DASH diet meal should be low in total fat, saturated fat, and cholesterol. However, to maintain balance in your diet, the DASH diet allows intake of fats, sweets, and red meat in small amounts. To help you plan your meal, I've listed the recommended servings for a 2,000-calorie diet from each food group.

- **Vegetables** – The recommended number of servings for vegetables per day is **4** to **5**.

It is highly recommended to incorporate vegetables that are high in magnesium, potassium, fiber, and other vitamins such as leafy green vegetables, sweet potatoes, broccoli, carrots, and tomatoes.

How to incorporate: If you want to fully benefit from vegetables, you can look for recipes that you can serve as a main dish such as the Bean Barley Burgers and Grilled California Veggie Sandwich. You can also serve fresh, frozen, or canned vegetables. However, when buying canned vegetables, always choose those without added salt or the low sodium variety.

- **Grains** – The recommended number of servings for grains per day is **6** to **8**.

Grains include pasta, rice, cereal, and bread. A single serving of grains can be ½ cup of pasta, rice or cereal or 1 slice of whole wheat bread. Whole grains have more nutrients and fiber compared to refined grain.

How to incorporate: Focus on taking whole grain variants like brown rice instead of white and whole wheat instead of regular pasta. Grains are normally low in fat so avoid serving it with cheese sauces, cream, and butter to keep it this way.

-     **Dairy** – The recommended number of servings for dairy per day is **2** to **3**.

Though dairy is usually a major source of fat, especially saturated fat, the DASH diet still recommends its intake because it is also a source of protein, Vitamin D, and calcium. Dairy products include cheese, yogurt, and milk but, to stay within the DASH diet threshold for fat intake, you should choose the fat-free or low fat variety. A single serving of dairy can be any of the following: 1 ½ ounces of part-skim cheese, 1 cup of low fat yogurt, or 1 cup skim milk.

How to incorporate: When craving for a sweet snack or dessert, just combine fruits with fat-free dairy products. Just go easy on cheeses because they also contain sodium. If you're lactose intolerant, you can opt for lactose-free dairy products so you can still include dairy into your diet. To prevent symptoms of lactose intolerance, there are over-the-counter medications available that contains "enzyme lactase" which effectively alleviates any unwanted indications.

-     **Fruits** – The recommended number of servings for fruits per day is **4** to **5**.

Fruits are also a good source of magnesium, potassium, and fiber and needs little to no preparation to add to a meal or become a healthy snack option. Like vegetables, fruits are also low in fat (except for coconuts) so you can take a few serving per day guiltlessly. A single serving of fruit can be 4 ounces of fresh juice, ½ cup of canned, fresh, or frozen fruit, or 1 medium fruit.

How to incorporate: To add meet your recommended daily servings for fruits, you can take one piece with meals and one as a treat. Or you can take it as a dessert of fresh mixed fruits with yogurt at the end of the day. Also, if the peels are edible, leave it on for more fiber and nutrients. Fruit skins also add interesting textures to different recipes. For canned fruits or juice, opt for the no-sugar-added varieties.

Note: Fruits and juices have citric acids that may not go well certain medications. If you need to take medicines regularly, contact your physician to check if you need to limit or avoid intake of certain fruits.

- **Fish, Poultry, and Lean Meat** – The recommended number of servings for fish, poultry, and lean meat per day is **6**.

For the DASH diet, a single serving of fish, poultry, or lean meat should be no more than 1 ounce. By cutting on meat, you can add more room for vegetables.

How to incorporate: When cooking meat and poultry, remove the skin and trim the fat. Cook by roasting, grilling, broiling, or baking instead of cooking in fat. When choosing fish, opt for the variety that is known to be good for the heart such as tuna, herring, and salmon. These kinds of fish can lower cholesterol because it contains Omega-3 fatty acids.

-        **Oils and Fats** – The recommended number of servings for oils and fats per day is **2** to **3**.

As we all know, fats have high caloric content and can cause problems associated with obesity, diabetes, and heart disease. However, fats are actually important components of diet. In fact, they can boost your body's immune system by enabling it to absorb essential nutrients and vitamins. The DASH diet allows for a limited intake of fat (up to 30% per day) to keep a healthy balance. A single serving of oils and fats can be 2 tablespoons of salad dressing, 1 tablespoon of mayonnaise, or 1 teaspoon of soft margarine.

How to incorporate: To avoid unhealthy fats, limit your intake of butter, eggs, meat, cream, whole milk and cheese. Also, avoid foods that are made with or contain palm or coconut oils, solid shortenings, and lard. Processed foods like fried items, baked goods, and crackers also contain trans-fat so avoid these as much as possible. If you're not sure which foods are low in saturated and trans fat, just check the food labels for content.

- **Legumes, Seeds, and Nuts** – The recommended number of servings for nuts, seeds, and legumes per week is **4** to **5**.

This type of foods is a good source of protein, potassium and magnesium. Examples of food belonging to this group are lentils, peas, kidney beans, sunflower seeds, and almonds. Aside from vitamins and nutrients, this food group also contains lots of fiber and phytochemicals that protects the body from cardiovascular disease and certain cancers. A single serving of nuts, seeds, and legumes can be ½ cup of cooked peas or beans, 2 tablespoons of seeds, or 1/3 cup of nuts.

How to incorporate: Nuts are high in calories and fats; that's why most diets restrict this type of food. However, they also contain Omega-3 fatty acids which are good for the heart. You can incorporate this type of food as toppings for cereals, salads, or stir-fries. You can also get your servings by replacing meat with soy products such as tempeh and tofu.

- **Sweets** – The recommended number of servings for sweets per week is **5** or less.

In order to keep a well-balanced diet, you should still allow a couple of servings of sweets into your system. A single serving of sweets can be 1 cup of lemonade, ½ cup of sorbet, or 1 tablespoon of jam or jelly.

How to incorporate: You can have cookies, crackers, hard candies, jelly beans, and sorbets if you're craving for sweet treats but it would be helpful if you choose the low-fat or fat-free variety over the regular ones. Also, when making desserts or sweet snacks, you can also use artificial sweeteners such as Splenda and Equal to minimize sugar intake.

The Effects of Caffeine and Alcohol

Too much alcohol intake can increase blood pressure. That's why DASH diet highlights the importance of setting a ceiling for alcohol intake. The maximum is 2 servings of alcohol per day for men and 1 serving per day for women. As for caffeine, its effect to blood pressure is still unclear as different people seem to have different levels of caffeine tolerance. If drinking caffeinated drinks causes your blood pressure to increase even temporarily, you must consult your doctor for proper recommendations.

DASH Diet and Losing Weight

Though DASH diet is not designed for weight loss, you may still lose some extra pounds due to healthier food choices and making your calories count. The standard DASH diet is set to provide you with 2,000 calories per day. If you want to lose weight, you can take fewer than the recommended calories however, make sure that you consult your doctor first as a sudden change in food intake may also trigger a harmful change in your blood pressure.

Cutting Back on Sodium Without Cutting Back on Flavor

Foods and meals promoted by the DASH diet are typically low in sodium but certainly don't lack in flavor. However, beginners may need some adjustment especially if they're used to strong and savory flavors. To help you gradually reduce your sodium intake, here are a few tips:

- Familiarize yourself with sodium-free flavorings and spices that you can use instead of salt.
- Rinse canned foods if possible to remove some of the added sodium.
- Avoid adding salt or other flavorings containing sodium when preparing cereal, pasta, or rice.
- Choose foods with labels such as "very low sodium", "low sodium", "sodium-free" or "no salt added" when buying in supermarkets.
- Get into the habit of reading food labels and you might be surprised how some foods have really high sodium content such as some canned soups, instant cereals, canned vegetables, and even the seemingly innocent sliced turkey from a local deli.

There is a noticeable difference between regular foods and the low-sodium variety. To give your palate some time to adjust, just cut back on using table salt and gradually introduce the lower sodium options to your meals. There are also some herb spice blends and other salt-free seasoning that may help ease the transition.

Starting Strong

Getting on any kind of diet can be difficult especially at the beginning. This is one of the main reasons that most people quit. The key to succeeding with the DASH diet is to learn to ease your way into your new food lifestyle. Below are some tips to help you do just that:

- **Allow yourself to adjust.** If you're not into vegetables and fruits or you need to majorly cut on your sweet treats, give yourself some time to adjust. Take baby steps by adding or removing a serving per day for each food group. While making changes on your diet, also note the changes you notice in your body whether positive or negative so you can pinpoint your problem areas (for example, you notice you get more gas when eating vegetables or beans or you get diarrhea when you eat grains). By knowing your problem areas, you'll be able to ask for advice from health professionals.

- **Add physical activities that you can manage.** A great way to get more positive results with your DASH diet is to add in more physical activities to help you lower your blood pressure. If your schedule permits you to exercise or go to the gym, do it. If not, you can also add more physical activities by walking or climbing the stairs more often. Don't push yourself to do more than you're capable of or your time allows.

- **Recognize your achievements and allow for slip-ups.** Reward your accomplishments with non-food treats like going out for a movie or purchasing new clothes (which might be a good idea since you're definitely going to lose some weight). Don't beat yourself up if you have a slip-up. Remember that changing habits takes quite a while. What you can do is to learn what triggered the setback and to just pick up where you left off.

-       **Don't be afraid to ask for support.** If you find it difficult to stick to the DASH diet, ask for help. Express your concerns with your dietitian or seek support from the DASH diet community.

CHAPTER 2

DASH Diet Recipes for Breakfast

Baked Apple-Spiced Oatmeal

Add a delicious twist to your everyday morning oatmeal.

Serves 9

Ingredients:

- ½ cup of sweetened applesauce
- 1 egg, beaten
- 1 teaspoon of vanilla
- 1 ½ cups of non-fat milk
- 1 ½ cups of chopped apple
- 2 tablespoons of oil
- 1 teaspoon of baking powder
- 2 cups of rolled oats
- 1 teaspoon of cinnamon
- ¼ teaspoon of salt

For the topping

- 2 tablespoons of chopped nuts
- 2 tablespoons of brown sugar

Directions:

1.	Set oven to 375F and preheat. Prepare an 8-inch square baking pan and lightly grease.

2.	Combine the milk, oil, vanilla, applesauce, and egg in a mixing bowl. Mix in the chopped apple. In another bowl, mix together the oats, cinnamon, salt, and baking powder. Add the oats mixture into the applesauce mixture and mix well until combined. Transfer the mixture into the prepared baking pan. Bake in the oven for 25 minutes.

3.	Once done, remove the baking pan from the oven and sprinkle the nuts and sugar on top. Broil in the oven for 4 minutes while keeping an eye to keep it from burning.

4.	Divide into 9 squares and serve while still warm.

Nutrition Info per Serving: **160 Calories, 6g Total Fat, 22g Carbohydrates, 6g Protein and 3g Fiber**

Applesauce French Toast

Your favorite French toast, only healthier.

Serves 6

Ingredients:

-	½ cup of milk

- 2 eggs
- 2 tablespoons of white sugar
- 1 teaspoon of ground cinnamon
- 6 slices of whole wheat bread
- ¼ cup of unsweetened applesauce

Directions:

1. Mix applesauce, sugar, cinnamon, milk, and eggs until thoroughly-combined.
2. Soak the bread, a piece at a time, until the mixture is absorbed slightly.
3. Set a lightly greased skillet over medium heat and cook the soaked bread slices until both sides are golden brown. Serve while still hot.

Nutrition Info per Serving: **150 Calories, 3g Total Fat, 27g Carbohydrates, 8g Protein and 2g Fiber**

Onion Asparagus Frittata

Get loaded every morning with this savory frittata.

Serves 4

Ingredients:

- 1 medium onion, sliced thinly
- 1 teaspoon of olive oil

- 2 cups of asparagus, cut into 1-inch pieces
- 2 teaspoons of balsamic vinegar
- ¼ cup of fresh basil, sliced thinly
- 3 green onions, sliced
- ¼ cup and 1 tablespoon of parmesan cheese, grated
- 6 large eggs
- Fresh ground pepper
- ½ teaspoon of kosher salt

Directions:

1. Set the broiler to high and preheat.

2. Set a 12-inch ovenproof skillet over medium heat. Add the olive oil. Once hot, add in the onions and cook for 5 minutes. Stir in the balsamic vinegar. Add 2 tablespoons of water and the asparagus. Cover with a lid and steam for 4 minutes.

3. Whisk the eggs and add in ¼ cup of the grated parmesan. Mix together until well-combined and season with ¼ teaspoon of kosher salt and freshly ground pepper.

4. Remove the lid from the skillet and add in the remaining kosher salt, basil, and green onions. Mix well.

5. Pour in the egg mixture into the skillet and stir briefly. Cook for 2 minutes.

6.   Place the skillet in the broiler and cook for 3 minutes. Once done, remove the skillet from the broiler and sprinkle the remaining parmesan on top. Rest for 5 minutes.

7.   Slice the frittata into 4 and serve immediately.

Nutrition Info per Serving: **190 Calories, 11g Total Fat, 8g Carbohydrates, 14g Protein and 2g Fiber**

Baked Sweet Potato

Enjoy a decadent anti-oxidant meal every morning.

Serves 1

Ingredients:

-     ½ tablespoon of butter, melted
-     1 small purple sweet potato
-     ¼ cup of blueberries
-     1/8 cup of crushed pecans
-     1 dash of cinnamon
-     ½ tablespoon of flaked coconut

Directions:

1.   Scrub clean the sweet potatoes under warm water. Pat dry and pierce several times with a fork.

2.   Wrap the sweet potato in a sheet of paper towel. Heat in the microwave for 3 ½ minutes. Rest for 5 minutes while still wrapped in paper towel.

3.   Melt the butter and slice open the sweet potato. Drizzle butter over the sweet potato and top with the cinnamon, blueberries, and pecans.

Nutrition Info per Serving: **297 Calories, 16g Total Fat, 37g Carbohydrates, 5g Protein and 5g Fiber**

Nutty Banana Pancakes

Hearty and delicious breakfast fit for the whole family.

Serves 6

Ingredients:

-      2 teaspoons of baking powder
-      1 cup of whole wheat flour
-      ¼ teaspoon of cinnamon
-      ¼ teaspoon of salt
-      1 cup of 1% milk
-      1 large banana, mashed
-      2 teaspoons of oil
-      3 large egg whites
-      2 tablespoons of chopped walnuts
-      1 teaspoon of vanilla

Directions:

1. Mix together the baking powder, flour, cinnamon, salt, and walnuts. Combine the mashed bananas, vanilla, oil, egg white, and milk in a separate bowl until smooth.

2. Pour the banana mixture into the flour mixture and mix together until well-combined. Be careful not to over-mix.

3. Set a large pan over medium heat. Lightly coat the pan with cooking spray. Pour ¼ cup of batter and cook until it starts to bubble. Flip and cook the other side. Do the same procedure with the remaining batter.

Nutrition Info per Serving: **146 Calories, 4g Total Fat, 22g Carbohydrates, 7g Protein and 3g Fiber**

Berry Morning Blast

This is a refreshingly delicious morning parfait for both kids and adults.

Serves 4

Ingredients:

- 1 cup of low fat granola
- 1 cup of rinsed strawberries, sliced
- 1 cup of low fat plain yogurt

-       1 cup of rinsed blueberries

Directions:

1.   Prepare 4 small glasses.

2.   Divide the strawberries equally between the 4 glasses. Sprinkle granola on top of the strawberries.

3.   Divide the blueberries equally between the 4 glasses and place on top of the granola. Spoon the yogurt on top of the blueberries and serve.

Nutrition Info per Serving: **150 Calories, 4g Total Fat, 27g Carbohydrates, 5g Protein and 3g Fiber**

Minty Morning Gazpacho

Serve a fruity gazpacho as an early morning treat for the whole family.

Serves 4

Ingredients:

-       1 ½ cups of raspberries
-       1 ½ cups of blueberries
-       1 tablespoon of orange juice
-       2 tablespoons of raw sugar
-       1 teaspoon of lime juice
-       1 teaspoon of lemon juice
-       Fresh mint leaves

- 1 teaspoon of lemon zest
- 1 cup of fat-free Greek yogurt

Directions:

1.   Mix lemon zest, lime juice, lemon juice, orange juice, sugar, raspberries and blueberries in a heatproof bowl. Cover the bowl tightly using a plastic wrap.

2.   Heat water in a large saucepan. Once simmering, set the covered bowl over the saucepan and cook for 10 minutes. Set aside to cool to room temperature. Refrigerate for 4 hours.

3.   Serve in bowls and top with fresh mint and ¼ cup of yogurt.

Nutrition Info per Serving: **112 Calories, 1g Total Fat, 23g Carbohydrates, 6g Protein and 4g Fiber**

Early Banana Split

Now, you can have dessert for breakfast.

Serves 2

Ingredients:

- ½ cup of oat cereal
- 1 small banana

- ½ teaspoon of honey
- ½ cup of low fat vanilla yogurt
- ½ cup of canned pineapple chunks

Directions:

1.   Peel the banana and halve lengthwise. Place each banana half in separate serving bowls.

2.   Sprinkle granola over the banana halves. Spoon yogurt on top of each and drizzle honey all over.

3.   Garnish with the pineapple chunks and sprinkle with extra granola on top. Serve immediately.

Nutrition Info per Serving: **180 Calories, 3.5g Total Fat, 34g Carbohydrates, 5g Protein and 3g Fiber**

Morning Bread Pudding

Nothing beats waking up to a warm and comfy bread pudding.

Serves 4

Ingredients:

- 4 eggs
- 1 ½ cups of low fat 1% milk
- ½ teaspoon of vanilla extract
- 2 tablespoons of brown sugar
- 1/8 teaspoon of salt

- ½ teaspoon of ground cinnamon
- ½ cup of peeled and diced apple
- 3 cups of cubed whole wheat bread
- 2 teaspoons of powdered sugar
- ¼ cup of raisins

Directions:

1. Set the oven to 350F and preheat.

2. Whisk together the salt, cinnamon, vanilla, brown sugar, eggs, and milk in a large bowl. Add in the raisins, apple, and bread cubes and mix together until well-combined and the bread has soaked up the liquid.

3. Prepare an 8-inch baking dish and coat with butter. Place the bread mixture into the prepared baking pan and cover with aluminum foil. Bake in the oven for 40 minutes. Remove the foil and bake for another 20 minutes.

4. Once done, set aside for 10 minutes. Dust with powdered sugar before serving.

Nutrition Info per Serving: **250 Calories, 6g Total Fat, 13g Protein and 3g Fiber**

Green Smoothie

Pack on nutrients early with this delicious green smoothie.

Serves 1

Ingredients:

- 1 cup of baby spinach, packed
- 1 medium banana
- ¼ cup of whole oats
- ½ cup of fat-free milk
- ¼ cup of non-fat plain yogurt
- ¾ cup of frozen mango
- ½ teaspoon of vanilla

Directions:

1. Mix together all the ingredients in a high-speed blender until smooth. Serve immediately.

Nutrition Info per Serving: **350 Calories, 2g Total Fat, 77g Carbohydrates, 12g Protein and 9g Fiber**

CHAPTER 3

DASH Diet Recipes for Main Dishes

Chicken Broccoli Stir-Fry

Skip Chinese and enjoy this healthy and hearty meal with the whole family.

Serves 4

Ingredients:

- 1 tablespoon of low sodium soy sauce
- 1/3 cup of orange juice
- 2 teaspoons of cornstarch
- 1 tablespoon of Szechuan sauce
- 1 lb of boneless chicken breast, cubed to 1-inch pieces
- 1 tablespoon of canola oil
- 6 oz of frozen snow peas
- 2 cups of frozen broccoli florets
- 2 cups of cooked brown rice
- 2 cups of shredded cabbage
- 1 tablespoon of sesame seeds

Directions:

1.   Combine the cornstarch, Szechuan sauce, soy sauce, and orange juice in a small bowl.

2.   Add the canola oil in a wok. Once the oil is hot, add in the chicken and stir fry for 7 minutes. Add in the snow peas, broccoli, cabbage, and the sauce mixture. Stir fry for 5 minutes.

3.   Serve on top of the brown rice. Sprinkle sesame seeds on top.

Nutrition Info per Serving: **340 Calories, 8g Total Fat, 35g Carbohydrates, 28g Protein and 5g Fiber**

Beef and Noodles

This is a must-try ramen noodle hack.

Serves 6

Ingredients:

-    ½ lb of lean ground beef

-    2 cups of water

-    1 pack of seasoning from the ramen-style noodles

-    2 packs of oriental instant ramen-style noodles, broken to little pieces

-    2 green onions, slice thinly

- 16 oz of frozen Asian-style vegetables
- 2 cloves of garlic, mince
- 1 tablespoon of fresh ginger

Directions:

1. Over medium-high heat, cook the ground beef in a large skillet until no longer pink. Drain the excess fat.

2. Add in the water and the seasoning packet and mix until well-combined.

3. Add in the garlic, ginger, green onion, and frozen vegetables. Mix together and bring the mixture to boil. Set the heat to high.

4. Reduce the heat to low and add in the ramen noodles. Simmer for 5 minutes while occasionally stirring.

Nutrition Info per Serving: **270 Calories, 10g Total Fat, 27g Carbohydrates, 17g Protein and 3g Fiber**

Quinoa Chicken Parmesan

This is a delicious and gluten-free main dish that is packed with protein.

Serves 6

Ingredients:

- 1 medium onion, dice
- 1 tablespoon of olive oil
- 2 tablespoons of balsamic vinegar
- 3 cloves of garlic, mince
- 15 oz of canned diced tomatoes
- 15 oz of canned tomato sauce
- 1 cup of quinoa
- Basil
- Oregano
- Pepper
- 1 lb of skinless and boneless chicken, cooked and cubed
- 2 cups of water
- 2 tablespoons of grated parmesan cheese
- 2/3 cup of shredded part-skim mozzarella cheese

Directions:

1. Set the oven to 375F and preheat. Prepare a 2-quart baking dish and spray with cooking oil.

2. To make the sauce, set a large skillet over medium heat. Add in the oil. Once hot, add in the onion and cook for 7 minutes while frequently stirring.

Add in the garlic and cook for 1 minute. Add in the balsamic vinegar and cook until most of the liquid is absorbed. Scrape any browned bits from the pan. Add in the pepper, oregano, basil, diced tomatoes, and tomato sauce. Stir together and bring the mixture to a low boil. Let simmer while preparing for the rest of the meal.

3.   To make the quinoa, rinse through a mesh strainer under cold water for 2 minutes. In a small saucepan, add in the water and quinoa. Bring to a boil then cover with a lid. Reduce heat and cook for 25 minutes.

4.   To serve, mix together the chicken and quinoa with the sauce until well-combined. Place the mixture in the prepared baking dish and sprinkle the mozzarella and parmesan on top. Bake in the oven for 10 minutes. Serve immediately.

Nutrition Info per Serving: **355 Calories, 10g Total Fat, 31g Carbohydrates, 33g Protein and 5g Fiber**

Bean Barley Burgers

Now you can have burgers for dinner.

Serves 8

Ingredients:

- 2 cups of kidney beans, cooked
- ½ teaspoon of garlic powder
- 1 tablespoon of olive oil
- ½ cup of wheat germ
- 3 cloves of garlic, mince
- ½ cup of onion, chop
- ½ teaspoon of sage
- 1 teaspoon of sea salt
- 2 cups of whole hull-less barley, cooked
- ½ teaspoon of celery seed, grind

Directions:

1. Mash the barley and beans together.
2. Fry the garlic and onion and add in to the mashed mixture together with the rest of the ingredients.
3. Form the mixture into 4-inch patties and cook over medium heat until both sides are browned.

Nutrition Info per Serving: **280 Calories, 4g Total Fat, 49g Carbohydrates, 12g Protein and 13g Fiber**

Beef with Pineapple Salsa

How does grilled beef sound for dinner?

Serves 6

Ingredients:

- Salt
- Pepper
- 1 ½ lbs of ranch steaks, 1-inch thick cut

For the marinade

- 2 tablespoons of olive oil
- 2 tablespoons of fresh lime juice
- 1 medium jalapeno pepper, mince
- 2 large cloves of garlic, mince
- ½ teaspoon of ground cumin

For the salsa

- 1 medium red onion, cut to make 12 wedges
- ½ medium pineapple, peel and cut to make 1 ½-inch chunks
- 2 teaspoons of lime zest

-      1 large red bell pepper, cut to make 1 ½-inch pieces

-      ½ teaspoon of salt

Directions:

1.   Mix together all the ingredients for the marinade in a medium bowl. Reserve 2 tablespoons. Cut the steaks to make 1 ¼-inch pieces and into the marinade. Toss until well-coated. Cover the bowl and let the beef marinate in the refrigerator for 30 minutes.

2.   Once done, remove the beef from the bowl and discard the marinade. Alternately thread the vegetable, fruit, and beef on 6 metal skewers.

3.   Over medium heat, grill the kabobs for 15 minutes while occasionally turning. Then, cover the grill and cook the kabobs for another 9 minutes while occasionally turning.

4.   Remove the grilled vegetables, fruit, and beef from the skewers. Chop the vegetables and fruit coarsely. Mix together the fruit and vegetables together with the salsa ingredients and reserved marinade. Season the beef with pepper and salt and serve with the salsa.

Nutrition Info per Serving: **207 Calories, 8g Total Fat, 9g Carbohydrates, 24g Protein and 1.5g Fiber**

Swiss Apple Panini

This is a crunchy sweet and salty sandwich blend that you'll want to eat over and over.

Serves 4

Ingredients:

- ¼ cup of non-fat honey mustard
- 8 slices of whole grain bread
- 6 oz of low fat Swiss cheese, slice thinly
- 2 crisp apples, slice thinly
- Cooking spray
- 1 cup of arugula leaves

Directions:

1. Spread the mustard evenly over the bread slices.
2. Layer the arugula leaves, cheese, and apple over 4 slices and top each with the remaining bread.
3. Grill each sandwich for 5 minutes in a Panini press or in a skillet. Once done, allow to slightly cool before serving.

Nutrition Info per Serving: **280 Calories, 4.5g Total Fat, 44g Carbohydrates, 17g Protein and 5g Fiber**

Grilled California Veggie Sandwich

Even meat-lovers will love this healthy veggie sandwich.

Serves 4

Ingredients:

- 3 cloves of garlic, mince
- 3 tablespoons of light mayonnaise
- 1/8 cup of olive oil
- 1 tablespoon of lemon juice
- 1 small zucchini, slice
- 1 cup of red bell peppers, slice
- 1 small yellow squash, slice
- 1 red onion, slice
- ½ cup of reduced-fat feta cheese, crumble
- 2 slices of focaccia bread

Directions:

1. Combine the lemon juice, garlic, and mayonnaise in a bowl. Place in the refrigerator until needed.
2. Set the grill to high heat and preheat.

3.   Coat the vegetables with olive oil and grease the grate. Place the zucchini and bell peppers near the center of the grill and place the squash and onions around the sides. Grill each side for 3 minutes.

4.   Spread mayonnaise over the cut side of the bread and sprinkle with crumbled feta. Grill the bread with the cheese side facing up for 2 minutes. Cover the grill with a lid. Once done, layer the vegetables on top of the bread slices and serve.

Nutrition Info per Serving: **240 Calories, 14g Total Fat, 24g Carbohydrates, 7g Protein and 2g Fiber**

Fresh Seafood Spring Rolls

This is a healthier option when you're craving for deep-fried spring rolls.

Serves 6

Ingredients:

-     12 bib lettuce leaves
-     12 sheets of rice paper
-     ¾ cup of fresh cilantro
-     12 basil leaves
-     ½ medium cucumber, slice thinly
-     1 cup of carrots, shredded

-        1 ¼ lbs of deveined and peeled shrimp, cooked

Directions:

1.   Dip a sheet of rice paper in warm water until just wet. Place on a clean cutting board.

2.   Layer 1 leaf of lettuce, 1 leaf of basil, and 1 tablespoon each of the cucumber, carrots, and cilantro. Place 4 shrimps over the vegetables and roll the rice paper like a burrito then tuck the ends. Repeat the procedure to make 12 fresh spring rolls.

3.   Serve immediately.

Nutrition Info per Serving: **180 Calories, 2g Total Fat, 17g Carbohydrates, 22g Protein and 1g Fiber**

Tuna Melt

Prepare a well-rounded lunch in 10 minutes.

Serves 4

Ingredients:

-        1/3 cup of chopped celery
-        6 oz of white tuna in water, drain
-        ¼ cup of low fat Russian salad dressing
-        ¼ cup of chopped onion
-        3 oz of reduced fat cheddar cheese, grate

- 2 whole wheat English muffins, split
- Salt
- Black pepper

Directions:

1. Preheat the broiler.

2. Mix together the salad dressing, onion, celery, and tuna. Taste and season accordingly with black pepper and salt. Toast the muffin halves. Place ¼ of the tuna mixture on each muffin halves and place on a baking dish. Broil for 3 minutes.

3. Top with the cheese and broil again for a minute.

Nutrition Info per Serving: **210 Calories, 6g Total Fat, 20g Carbohydrates, 19g Protein and 3g Fiber**

Tuna Salad

Experience a nice change from the traditional tuna salads.

Serves 2

Ingredients:

- 1 tablespoon of extra-virgin olive oil
- 5 oz of canned tuna in water, drain
- ¼ cup of chopped green onion

- 1 tablespoon of red wine vinegar
- 1 cup of cooked pasta
- 2 cups of arugula
- Black pepper
- 1 tablespoon of freshly shaved parmesan cheese

Directions:

1.   Mix together all of the ingredients in a salad bowl except for the pepper and parmesan. Once well-combined, season with pepper and top with cheese. Serve immediately.

Nutrition Info per Serving: **245 Calories, 7g Total Fat, 23g Carbohydrates, 23g Protein and 1g Fiber**

DASH Diet Recipes for Desserts

Almond Rice Pudding

This treat is tasty, healthy, and guilt-free.

Serves 6

Ingredients:

- 1 cup of white rice
- 3 cups of 1% milk
- 1 teaspoon of vanilla
- ¼ cup of sugar
- Cinnamon
- ¼ teaspoon of almond extract
- ¼ cup of toasted almonds

Directions:

1. Mix together the rice and milk in a saucepan and bring the mixture to boil.
2. Reduce the heat and simmer for 30 minutes covered.

3.　　Once done, remove the saucepan from the heat and add in the cinnamon, almond extract, vanilla, and sugar. Mix well.

4.　　Sprinkle toasted almonds before serving.

Nutrition Info per Serving: **180 Calories, 1.5g Total Fat, 36g Carbohydrates, 7g Protein, and 1g Fiber**

Creamy Apple Shake

Make this calcium-rich dessert in less than 10 minutes.

Serves 4

Ingredients:

- 1 cup of unsweetened applesauce
- 2 cups of low fat vanilla ice cream
- 1 cup of fat-free skim milk
- ¼ teaspoon of ground cinnamon

Directions:

1. Mix together all of the ingredients in a blender and pour into glasses.
2. Top with extra cinnamon and serve.

Nutrition Info per Serving: **160 Calories, 3g Total Fat, 27g Carbohydrates, 6g Protein and 1g Fiber**

Baked Apples

Try this recipe that can warm you up on cold days.

Serves 4

Ingredients:

- ¼ cup of flaked coconut

- 4 Golden Delicious apples
- 2 teaspoons of grated orange zest
- ¼ cup of chopped dried apricots
- 2 tablespoons of brown sugar
- ½ cup of orange juice

Directions:

1. Peel the apples and remove the core by hollowing out the center. Arrange on a heatproof baking dish. Mix together the orange zest, apricots, and coconuts until well-combined. Fill the apples with the mixture evenly.

2. Combine the brown sugar and orange juice. Pour the mixture over the apples. Cover the baking dish tightly with a plastic wrap. Poke the wrap to create vents. Microwave on high settings for 8 minutes.

Nutrition Info per Serving: **192 Calories, 2g Total Fat, 46g Carbohydrates, 1g Protein and 6g Fiber**

Orange Rice Pudding

Creamy orangey vanilla pudding that will make every morning a treat!

Serves 6

Ingredients:

- 3 large navel oranges
- ¾ cup of basmati rice
- 4 cups of fat-free evaporated milk
- ½ vanilla bean, halve lengthwise
- 4 tablespoons of sugar
- ¼ cup of low fat and sweetened condensed milk
- 2 tablespoons of pomegranate seeds
- 2 tablespoons of chopped pistachios

Directions:

1. Add 2 cups of water in a saucepan and bring to boil. Add in the rice and reduce the heat. Cover the saucepan with a lid and simmer the rice for 20 minutes.

2. Take 1 teaspoon of zest from one of the oranges. Juice the orange and reserve.

3. Segment the remaining oranges by removing the rind, pith, and the membrane. Set the segments aside.

4. Add ½ cup of the orange juice to the rice once it's tender. Stir in the orange zest, sugar, condensed milk, evaporated milk, and vanilla bean.

5.   Cook the rice for another 25 minutes uncovered while stirring frequently until the pudding has is creamy in consistency.

6.   Remove the vanilla bean and serve. Top with the pomegranate seeds and pistachios.

Nutrition Info per Serving: **286 Calories, 2g Total Fat, 52g Carbohydrates, 16g Protein and 2g Fiber**

Berry Healthy Popsicles

This dessert is full of nutrients -- and perfect for hot summer afternoons.

Serves 8

Ingredients:

-       1 cup of blackberries
-       1 cup of blueberries
-       1 ¼ cups of non-fat milk
-       1 cup of non-fat plain yogurt

Directions:

1.   Mix together all the ingredients in a blender until well-combined. Pour ½ cup of the mixture into each popsicle mold and freeze for half an hour.

2.   Insert popsicle sticks then freeze for another 1 hour.

Nutrition Info per Serving: **47 Calories, 0g Total Fat, 9g Carbohydrates, 3g Protein and 1g Fiber**

Nutty Oat Blackberry Crumble

Summer berry plus sweet nuts and oats is a medley made in heaven.

Serves 4

Ingredients:

- 1 tablespoon of cornstarch
- 2 tablespoons of sugar
- ½ teaspoon of lemon juice
- 2 cups of fresh blackberries
- ¼ cup of all-purpose flour
- ½ cup of rolled oats
- ½ teaspoon of cinnamon
- ¼ cup of brown sugar
- 1 tablespoon of unsalted butter, dice
- 1/8 teaspoon of salt

-       ¼ cup of hazelnuts, chop

Directions:

1.   Set the oven to 350F and preheat. Prepare an 8-inch baking dish and coat with cooking spray.

2.   Mix together the sugar, cornstarch, blackberries, and lemon juice until well-combined. Place the mixture into the prepared baking dish.

3.   In another bowl, mix together the salt, cinnamon, brown sugar, flour, and oats. Add in the butter and stir until the mixture is sandy and crumbly in consistency. Stir in the nuts. Sprinkle the crumble on top of the berries.

4.   Bake for 30 minutes and serve while still warm.

Nutrition Info per Serving: **240 Calories, 8g Total Fat, 39g Carbohydrates, 4g Protein and 6g Fiber**

Blueberry Delight

This is a dessert you can enjoy year-round.

Serves 4

Ingredients:

- 2 teaspoons of soft salted butter
- 3 cups of fresh blueberries
- 1 tablespoon of brown sugar
- 1 tablespoon of all-purpose flour
- ½ teaspoon of cinnamon
- ½ cup of rolled oats

Directions:

1. Set the oven to 375F and preheat.

2. Prepare a 9-inch pie plate. Rinse and dry the blueberries and place it in the prepared pie plate.

3. Mix together the cinnamon, oats, sugar, flour, and butter. Sprinkle the mixture over the blueberries and bake for 25 minutes.

4. Serve warm.

Nutrition Info per Serving: **140 Calories, 3g Total Fat, 28g Carbohydrates, 3g Protein and 4g Fiber**

California Skinny Dips

Enjoy strawberries with three delicious dips.

Serves 6

Ingredients:

- 4 ½ cups of fresh strawberries

For the strawberry crème dip

- ¼ cup of strawberries
- ½ cup of reduced fat sour cream
- Strawberry jam

For the choco fudge dip

- 6 tablespoons of chocolate fudge sauce
- 6 tablespoons of non-fat yogurt
- 1 ½ teaspoons of orange juice concentrate

For the almond honey dip

- 3 tablespoons of toasted almonds, chop
- 2/3 cup of non-fat yogurt
- 2 ½ tablespoons of honey

Directions:

1. Wash the strawberries then pat dry.
2. To make each dip, just whisk together the ingredients until smooth then place in separate bowls.
3. Serve strawberries with the dips.

Nutrition Info per Serving: **200 Calories, 4g Total Fat, 39g Carbohydrate, 4g Protein and 3g Fiber**

Dark Chocolate Parfait

This is a rich probiotic snack unlike any other.

Serves 1

Ingredients:

- 1 tablespoon of miniature dark chocolate chips
- 2/3 cup of plain low fat kefir
- ½ cup of frozen banana
- 1 tablespoon of shredded unsweetened coconut

Directions:

1. Thaw the banana for 30 minutes and slice.
2. Place the kefir in a bowl and sprinkle with the coconut, chocolate chips and banana slices. Serve immediately.

Nutrition Info per Serving: **220 Calories, 9g Total Fat, 30g Carbohydrates, 8g Protein, 9g Fiber**

Apple Cranberry Risotto Dessert

If you haven't tried Risotto for dessert, this recipe is a must-try.

Serves 4

Ingredients:

- 3 ½ cups of fat-free milk
- ½ cup of dried cranberries
- 1 pinch of salt
- 1 cinnamon stick
- 1 large Golden Delicious apple, peel and core then dice to make 1 ½ cups
- 1 tablespoon of butter
- 1 ½ cups of apple cider
- ½ cup of Arborio rice
- 1 teaspoon of vanilla
- 2 tablespoons of packed light brown sugar

Directions:

1. Place the cranberries in a bowl and cover with boiling water. Let sit for 30 minutes.

2. Heat the salt, cinnamon stick, and milk in the microwave. Set aside and cover until needed.

3. In a Dutch oven set over medium heat, add in the butter. Once melted, add in the diced apple and cook for 2 minutes while frequently stirring. Add in

the rice and cook for 30 seconds. Add in ¾ cup of the apple cider and cook for 2 minutes. Add the remaining apple cider and cook again until most of the liquid has evaporated. Add in the sugar and mix well.

4.   Add ½ cup of warm milk and the cinnamon stick into the Dutch oven and cook for 3 minutes while frequently stirring.

5.   Add the remaining milk and cook for 20 minutes. The risotto should be creamy in consistency at this point. Once done, remove from the risotto from the heat and discard the cinnamon stick.

6.   Drain the cranberries and mix into the risotto together with the vanilla. Cool for 10 minutes before serving.

Nutrition Info per Serving: **336 Calories, 4g Total Fat, 71g Carbohydrates, 9g Protein, 3g Fiber**

CHAPTER 5

DASH Diet Recipes for Snacks

Fiber-Rich Apple Bran Muffins

Try these homemade muffins that are both low in fat and cholesterol, not to mention yummy and delicious.

Serves 12

Ingredients:

- ¾ cup of whole wheat flour
- ¾ cup of all-purpose flour
- 1 teaspoon of baking powder
- 1 ½ teaspoons of cinnamon
- ¼ teaspoon of salt
- ½ teaspoon of baking soda
- ½ cup of oat bran
- 1 cup of buttermilk
- 2 tablespoons of vegetable oil
- ¼ cup of firmly packed brown sugar
- 1 ½ cups of chopped Golden Delicious apples
- 1 large egg

Directions:

1.   Set the oven to 400F and preheat.

2.   Prepare a 12-cup muffin tin and line with paper liners.

3.   Mix together the salt, baking soda, baking powder, cinnamon, all-purpose flour, and whole wheat flour in a bowl.

4.   In another bowl, beat together the egg, oil, brown sugar, oat bran, and buttermilk. Pour the wet mixture into the dry mixture and stir until just combined. Fold in the apples.

5.   Pour the batter into the prepared muffin cups and bake for 20 minutes. Cool for 5 minutes then transfer to a wire rack to cool completely.

Nutrition Info per Serving: **121 Calories, 3g Total Fat, 21g Carbohydrates, 4g Protein and 3g Fiber**

Blueberry Muffins

These tasty snacks are good enough for breakfast or dessert.

Serves 12

Ingredients:

- ½ cup of old-fashioned whole oatmeal
- 1 ½ cups of flour
- ½ teaspoon of baking powder
- 1/3 cup of sugar
- ½ teaspoon of salt
- ¼ teaspoon of baking soda
- ½ cup of dry milk
- 1 cup of milk
- 1 egg
- ¼ cup of oil
- 2/3 cup of frozen blueberries

Directions:

1.   Turn on the oven and set to 350F and preheat. Prepare a 12-cup muffin tin and grease with cooking spray.

2.   Mix together the salt, baking soda, baking powder, sugar, oatmeal, and flour in a bowl. In a separate bowl, combine the egg, oil, dry milk, and milk.

3.   Stir together the dry and wet mixture. Add the blueberries and mix gently. The batter should still be lumpy at this point. Scoop into the prepared muffin tins and bake for 20 minutes. Serve warm.

Nutrition Info per Serving: **150 Calories, 5g Fat, 22g Carbohydrates, 4g Protein, and 1g Fiber**

Crispy Garbanzo

Enjoy savory beans for a healthy snack.

Serves 8

Ingredients:

- ½ teaspoon of salt
- 2 (15 oz) cans of unsalted garbanzo beans
- 1 teaspoon of garlic powder
- ½ teaspoon of pepper
- 1 teaspoon of dried parsley flakes
- 1 teaspoon of onion powder
- 2 teaspoons of dried dill

Directions:

1.   Set the oven to 400F and preheat.
2.   Drain the canned garbanzo beans and pat dry with paper towel.
3.   Mix together the dill, parsley, onion powder, garlic powder, pepper, and salt in a small bowl.

4.   Grease a rimmed baking sheet and spread the garbanzo beans on top. Spray the beans with cooking spray and sprinkle the seasoning mixture over the beans. Shake the baking sheet to coat the beans evenly with the seasoning. Spread the beans into a single layer. Bake for 40 minutes. Cool before serving.

Nutrition Info per Serving: **111 Calories, 1g Total Fat, 20g Carbohydrates, 6g Protein and 4g Fiber**

Fresh Melon Cooler

This is a refreshing melon cooler full of Vitamin C.

Serves 3

Ingredients:

- 1 cup of low-fat lemon yogurt
- 2 cups of cubed cantaloupe
- 1 cup of orange juice

Directions:

1.   Mix all the ingredients in a blender until smooth. Serve immediately.

Nutrition Info per Serving: **120 Calories, 1g Total Fat, 22g Carbohydrates, 5g Protein and 1g Fiber**

Lemony Berry Oatmeal Muffins

These spring treats are especially made for DASH dieters.

Serves 12

Ingredients:

- 2 tablespoons of firmly packed brown sugar
- 1 ¾ cups of old-fashioned oats
- ½ cup of granulated sugar
- 1 cup + 2 tablespoons of all-purpose flour
- ¼ teaspoon of salt
- 1 tablespoon of baking powder
- 2 egg whites, beaten lightly
- 1 cup of fat-free milk
- 1 teaspoon of lemon zest
- 2 tablespoons of vegetable oil
- 1 cup of fresh blueberries
- 1 teaspoon of vanilla

Directions:

1.   Set the oven to 400F and preheat. Prepare a 12-cup muffin tin and line with paper cups.

2.   Mix together the brown sugar and ¼ cup of oats to make the topping. Set aside until needed.

3.   To make the muffins, combine the rest of the ingredients and fill the muffin cups up to ¾ of the way. Sprinkle the toppings then bake for 24 minutes. Cool for 5 minutes before serving.

Nutrition Info per Serving: **160 Calories, 3g Total Fat, 33g Carbohydrates, 4g Protein and 2g Fiber**

Energizing Lemon Smoothie

This treat is especially refreshing and satisfying after an afternoon of workout.

Serves 1

Ingredients:

- 6 oz of fat-free plain yogurt
- 3 milk ice cubes, cracked
- 1 teaspoon of fresh lemon juice
- 2 tablespoons of granulated sugar

- ½ teaspoon of finely grated lemon zest

Directions:

1. Mix together all of the ingredients in a blender until smooth. Pour into a serving glass and enjoy!

Nutrition Info per Serving: **190 Calories, 1g Total Fat, 36g Carbohydrates, 13g Protein and 0g Fiber**

Pumpkin Bread

This flavorful bread is perfect in the fall or winter.

Serves 8

Ingredients:

- ¾ cup of low fat milk
- 1 cup of pumpkin puree
- 2 eggs
- 1 cup of sugar
- ½ teaspoon of baking powder
- 2 cups of whole wheat pastry flour
- ¼ teaspoon of ground cloves
- 1 teaspoon of baking soda
- 1 teaspoon of ground allspice
- 1 teaspoon of ground cinnamon

-      ¼ teaspoon of ground nutmeg

Directions:

1.   Set the oven to 350F and preheat. Prepare a loaf pan and grease with butter. Dust with flour and set aside until needed.

2.   Whisk together the milk, pumpkin puree, eggs, and sugar in a bowl. Add in the baking powder, pastry flour, cloves, baking soda, allspice, cinnamon, and nutmeg and mix until well-combined.

3.   Pour the batter into the loaf pan and bake for 55 minutes. Cool for 15 minutes in the pan before transferring on a wire rack to cool completely.

Nutrition Info per Serving: **240 Calories, 2g Total Fat, 51g Carbohydrates, 6g Protein and 5g Fiber**

Powerhouse Morning Muffins

This morning snack is full of calcium and protein and goes perfectly well with a fat-free latte or a glass of milk.

Serves 12

Ingredients:

-      1 cup of low fat milk

- 1 egg
- 2 tablespoons of vegetable oil
- 1/3 cup of sugar
- ½ cup of raisins
- ½ cup of grated carrots
- 1 teaspoon of vanilla
- ½ cup of toasted walnuts
- 1 cup of old-fashioned oatmeal
- 1 ½ cups of flour
- 1 teaspoon of baking powder
- 1 teaspoon of cinnamon
- ½ teaspoon of salt
- ½ teaspoon of baking soda

Directions:

1. Set the oven to 400F and preheat. Prepare a 12-cup muffin tin and grease with cooking spray.

2. Mix together the vanilla, walnuts, raisins, carrots, vegetable oil, sugar, milk and egg until well-combined.

3. In another bowl, mix together the salt, baking soda, baking powder, cinnamon, oatmeal, and flour. Pour the egg mixture into the bowl and stir gently until just combined. Fill the prepared muffin cups with the batter about ¾ of the way.

4. Bake in the oven for 15 minutes.

Nutrition Info per Serving: **180 Calories, 6g Total Fat, 26g Carbohydrates, 4g Protein and 2g Fiber**

Fruit Lassi

This refreshing wintry smoothie is rich in calcium and can also be taken as breakfast or light dessert.

Serves 2

Ingredients:

- ½ medium ripe banana
- 1 cup of fresh peaches
- 1 cup of low fat buttermilk
- ½ cup of fresh raspberries
- 3 ice cubes

Directions:

1. Mix all the ingredients together in a blender until smooth enough for drinking. Serve immediately.

Nutrition Info per Serving: **120 Calories, 0.5g Total Fat, 24g Carbohydrates, 5g Protein and 4g Fiber**

Power Smoothie

This is a kid-friendly spinach treat.

Serves 4

Ingredients:

- ½ cup of pineapple juice
- 1 cup of orange juice
- 1 banana, peel and slice
- ½ cup of low fat plain yogurt
- Crushed ice
- 2 cups of fresh spinach leaves

Directions:

1. Mix all the ingredients together in a blender until smooth enough for drinking. Serve immediately.

Nutrition Info per Serving: **93 Calories, 1g Total Fat, 204g Carbohydrates, 2g Protein and 2g Fiber**

CHAPTER 6

DASH Diet Recipes for Soup

Autumn Stew

This is a colorful homemade stew that will save you from high sodium canned soups and supply you with fiber and antioxidants.

Serves 6

Ingredients:

- 1 medium onion, chop
- 3 tablespoons of olive oil
- 2 ½ cups of peeled and cubed acorn squash
- 2 cloves of garlic, mince
- 1 fresh jalapeno, remove seeds and dice
- 1 ½ cups of green beans, slice to make 2-in pieces
- 14 oz of no-salt-added diced tomatoes
- 1 cup of corn kernels
- ½ tablespoon of white wine vinegar
- ½ cup of low sodium vegetable stock

Directions:

1.   Heat the olive oil in a skillet set over medium heat. Add in the garlic and onion and sauté until the onion softens.

2.   Add in the jalapeno, green beans, and squash. Cook for another 5 minutes. Add the rest of the ingredients and cover the skillet. Reduce temperature to medium-low. Simmer the soup for 30 minutes. Serve while still warm.

Nutrition Info per Serving: **170 Calories, 7g Total Fat, 25g Carbohydrates, 3g Protein and 6g Fiber**

Fennel Apple Soup

Enjoy this low sodium, low fat, creamy and smooth soup -- perfect for lunch or dinner.

Serves 4

Ingredients:

-       2 cups of water
-       14.5 oz of low sodium chicken broth
-       2 Golden Delicious apples, peel and core then chop

- ½ cup of white wine
- 1 small onion, slice thinly
- 1 cup of thinly sliced carrots
- 1 bay leaf
- ½ cup of chopped fresh fennel
- 6 black peppercorns
- ¼ teaspoon of dried thyme leaves
- Low fat plain yogurt

Directions:

1.   Mix together all the ingredients in a large pot. Cook until boiling then reduce the heat. Cover the pot with a lid and simmer for 20 minutes.

2.   Remove the bay leaf and pour the soup over a strainer. Reserve the liquid and puree the vegetables until smooth. Return the puree into the pot and add in the reserved liquid. Heat the soup before serving. Top each serving with yogurt.

Nutrition Info per Serving: **109 Calories, 1g Total Fat, 20g Carbohydrates, 2g Protein and 3g Fiber**

Ginger Squash Bisque

Support cell growth and care for your vision with this cozy and warm soup.

Serves 5

Ingredients:

- 2 cups of sliced onions
- 2 teaspoons of vegetable oil
- 2 pears, peel and core then dice
- 2 lbs of winter squash, peel and deseed then cut to make 2-inch cubes
- 2 tablespoons of coarsely chopped and peeled ginger
- 2 cloves of garlic, peel and crush
- 4 cup of low sodium chicken broth
- ½ teaspoon of thyme
- 1 tablespoon of lemon juice
- 1 cup of water
- ½ cup of non-fat plain yogurt

Directions:

1. Heat the vegetable oil in a pot set over medium heat. Add in the onions and sauté for 4 minutes. Add

in the thyme, ginger, garlic, pears, and squash and cook for a minute while stirring continuously.

2.   Add in the water and broth then bring the mixture to simmer. Reduce the temperature to low. Cover the pot with a lid and simmer for 45 minutes.

3.   Puree the soup in a blender until smooth. Once done, return the pureed soup into the pot to heat through. Stir in the lemon juice. Serve each serving with yogurt on top.

Nutrition Info per Serving: **173 Calories, 2g Total Fat, 38g Carbohydrates, 4g Protein and 7g Fiber**

Beef Barley Soup

This savory dish packed with vegetables will help you meet your daily nutrition needs.

Serves 14

Ingredients:

-     1 medium carrot, diced

- 1 lb of lean ground beef
- 1 stalk of celery, diced
- 1 medium onion, diced
- 1 cup of barley
- 2 cloves of garlic, chop finely
- 1 cup of low sodium beef bouillon
- 8 cups of water
- ½ teaspoon of pepper
- 14.5 oz of unsalted diced tomatoes in juice

Directions:

1.   Cook the ground beef in a large pot set over medium heat.

2.   Add in the garlic, celery, onion, and carrots and cook for 5 minutes while stirring often.

3.   Add in the water, barley, tomatoes with its juices, and the beef bouillon. Stir then bring the soup to boil. Cover the pot with a lid then reduce the temperature to low. Simmer for 40 minutes. Season with pepper and serve.

Nutrition Info per Serving: **110 Calories, 1.5g Total Fat, 16g Carbohydrates, 9g Protein and 3g Fiber**

Pear and Butternut Squash Soup

This is a slightly sweet and creamy soup perfect for any time of the day.

Serves 8

Ingredients:

- 1 lb of fresh pears, cored then cut to make 1/2-inch cubes
- 1 lb of butternut squash, cut to make ½-inch cubes
- ¼ teaspoon of salt
- 2 tablespoons of vegetable oil
- 2 tablespoons of butter
- ¼ teaspoon of black pepper
- 2 teaspoons of ground ginger
- 1 large onion, sliced thinly
- 8 oz of reduced fat sour cream
- 32 oz of reduced sodium vegetable broth

Directions:

1. Set the oven to 400F.
2. Place the squash and pears in a large bowl. Add in the oil, salt and black pepper. Toss together until both squash and pears are well-coated with oil and seasoned evenly. Place the squash and pears on a

baking sheet and spread in a single layer. Roast the vegetables in the oven for 30 minutes.

3.   Set a large pot over medium-low heat and melt the butter. Add in the onion and sauté for 10 minutes. Add in the ginger and stir. Cook for 1 minute. Remove the pot from the heat until the vegetables are done roasting.

4.   Add the roasted pears and squash into the pot and pour in the broth. Set the pot over medium-high heat and bring the soup to boil. Reduce the temperature then simmer for 10 minutes.

5.   Puree the soup in a blender until smooth. Return to the pot and simmer. Then, stir in the sour cream and season with pepper and salt before serving.

Nutrition Info per Serving: **210 Calories, 9g Total Fat, 32g Carbohydrates, 3g Protein and 6g Fiber**

Gazpacho Topped with Cilantro Yogurt

This chilled soup topped with infused yogurt will keepyou cool during summers.

Serves 4

Ingredients:

- ½ cup of chopped fresh cilantro
- 2 cups of fat-free plain yogurt
- 1 large red bell pepper
- 4 large tomatoes
- 1 large onion, chop
- 2 medium cucumbers, peel and deseed then slice
- ¼ cup of red wine vinegar
- 3 cups of tomato juice
- ¼ teaspoon of pepper
- 2 teaspoons of red pepper sauce
- 1 clove of garlic, chop finely

Directions:

1. Mix together the cilantro and 1 cup of yogurt then set aside until needed.
2. Add the remaining yogurt, bell pepper, tomatoes, onion, cucumbers, and onion in a blender until smooth and well-combined.
3. Add the remaining ingredients and process until well-incorporated. Refrigerate the soup for 2 hours and serve with the cilantro yogurt on top.

Nutrition Info per Serving: **190 Calories, 0.5g Total Fat, 38g Carbohydrates, 12g Protein and 6g Fiber**

Turkey Chili

Try this quick-cooking chili with the smokiness of peppers and cumin.

Serves 6

Ingredients:

- 2 tablespoons of diced onion
- 1 tablespoon of olive oil
- 15 oz of canned low sodium black beans
- 2 teaspoons of diced garlic
- 3 tablespoons of roasted red pepper in water, drained
- 1 cup of shredded pre-cooked turkey
- ½ tablespoon of chili powder
- 32 oz of canned roasted diced tomato in juice
- ½ teaspoon of red pepper flakes
- 1 tablespoon of cumin
- 6 tablespoons of fat-free plain yogurt
- ½ teaspoon of salt
- 6 tablespoons of shredded cheddar cheese

Directions:

1.	Heat the olive oil in a Dutch oven set over medium heat. Add in the garlic and onions and sauté for 4 minutes. Add the remaining ingredients except for the cheese and yogurt. Stir until combined. Cover with a lid and simmer for 15 minutes.

2.	Serve with cheese and yogurt on top.

Nutrition Info per Serving: **140 Calories, 4g Total Fat, 16g Carbohydrates, 11g Protein and 5g Fiber**

Lentil Chili

Enjoy this fiber-rich vegetarian soup alternative.

Serves 6

Ingredients:

-	1 onion, chop
-	2 tablespoons of vegetable oil
-	1 cup of dry lentils
-	4 cloves of garlic, mince
-	3 cups of low sodium and low fat chicken broth
-	1 cup of dry bulgur wheat

- 2 tablespoons of chili powder
- 2 cups of canned whole tomatoes, chop
- Salt
- Pepper
- 1 tablespoon of ground cumin

Directions:

1. Add the vegetable oil, garlic, and onion in a pot set on medium-high heat. Cook for 5 minutes. Stir in the bulgur wheat and lentils. Add in the pepper, salt, cumin, chili powder, tomatoes, and broth. Bring the soup to boil then reduce the temperature to low. Simmer for another 30 minutes.

Nutrition Info per Serving: **281 Calories, 6g Total Fat, 45g Carbohydrates, 14g Protein and 17g Fiber**

Fresh Mushroom Soup

This is a creamy and delicious soup you can enjoy guiltlessly.

Serves 4

Ingredients:

- 1 cup of diced carrots
- 2 teaspoons of butter
- 1 teaspoon of minced garlic
- ½ cup of thinly sliced scallions
- ¼ teaspoon of ground black pepper
- ¼ teaspoon of dried thyme
- 14.5 oz of low sodium vegetable broth
- 1 ½ lbs of white mushrooms, sliced
- 1 ½ cups of low fat milk
- 1 cup of white wine

Directions:

1.   Melt the butter in a saucepan set over medium-high heat. Add in the garlic, onions, carrots, pepper, and thyme and sauté for 5 minutes. Add in the wine, broth, and mushrooms then bring the mixture to boil. Cook for 1 minute. Remove 1 cup of the vegetables and set it aside.

2.   Puree the soup in a blender until smooth. Return the soup into the saucepan and stir in the reserved vegetables and milk. Simmer for 5 minutes. Serve and top with extra chopped scallions on top.

Nutrition Info per Serving: **120 Calories, 3.5g Total Fat, 15g Carbohydrates, 10g Protein and 3g Fiber**

Mushroom Chili

This hearty chili can be perfectly paired with fresh cut sticks of veggies and whole grain crackers.

Serves 4

Ingredients:

- 1 cup of chopped onion
- 2 tablespoons of vegetable oil
- 2 tablespoons of chili powder
- 1 tablespoon of minced garlic
- 1 ½ lbs of white button mushrooms, sliced
- 1 teaspoon of ground cumin
- 14.5 oz of stewed tomatoes
- 8 oz of shiitake mushrooms, sliced
- ½ cup of sliced ripe olives
- 19 oz of white kidney beans, rinse and drain

Directions:

1. Heat the vegetable oil in a saucepan. Add in the garlic and onion and cook for 5 minutes. Stir in the cumin and chili powder and cook for 30 seconds. Add in the mushrooms and cook for 8 minutes.

2.   Add in ½ cup of water, olives, beans, and the stewed tomatoes into the saucepan. Simmer uncovered for 10 minutes.

3.   Serve with whole grain tortillas and top with shredded cheddar, lettuce, and diced tomatoes.

Nutrition Info per Serving: **300 Calories, 10g Total Fat, 45g Carbohydrates, 12g Protein and 10g Fiber**

CHAPTER 7

DASH Diet Recipes for Salads

Chicken Almond Pear Salad

This is a healthy chicken salad that can be also made into a sandwich using whole wheat bread.

Serves 4

Ingredients:

- ½ cup of green pepper, slice lengthwise
- 2 cups of cooked skinless and boneless chicken breasts, cut to make ½-inch cubes
- ¼ teaspoon of salt
- ¼ cup of diced celery
- 2 tablespoons of reduced-calorie mayonnaise
- ½ cup of low fat plain yogurt
- ¼ teaspoon of ground ginger
- ½ teaspoon of prepared mustard
- Lettuce
- 2 Bosc pears, cored and cut to make 1-inch cubes
- 2 tablespoons of toasted slivered almonds

Directions:

1.   Toss together the celery, green pepper, and chicken. Season with salt.

2.   In a separate bowl, mix together the ginger, mustard, mayonnaise, and yogurt until well-combined. Add the dressing into the chicken mixture and gently stir in the pears. Mix together until well-coated. Serve over lettuce leaves and top with almonds.

Nutrition Info per Serving: **232 Calories, 7g Total Fat, 18g Carbohydrates, 24g Protein and 4g Fiber**

Mango Amaranth Salad

This beautiful and delicious grain salad is perfect for picnics and summer potlucks.

Serves 4

Ingredients:

- 1 ½ teaspoons of curry powder
- ½ cup of plain yogurt

- 1 cup of amaranth grain, uncooked
- 1 teaspoon of ginger, grated
- 1 ½ cups of mango, chop
- 1 ½ cups of water
- 1 cup of low sodium canned black beans, drain and rinse
- ½ cup of red bell pepper, dice
- 1 tablespoon of fresh mint
- 1 tablespoon of jalapeno, dice
- 2 tablespoons of cilantro, chop

Directions:

1. Mix together the ginger, curry powder, and yogurt in a bowl and refrigerate until needed.

2. Add the water in a medium saucepan and bring to boil. Add in the amaranth and reduce the temperature to low. Simmer for 25 minutes. Remove the saucepan from the heat and drain the excess liquid.

3. Toss together the amaranth, herbs, jalapeno, black beans, bell pepper, and mango. Add in the chilled dressing and mix together until well-coated. Chill before serving.

Nutrition Info per Serving: **320 Calories, 4g Total Fat, 63g Carbohydrates, 11g Protein and 9g Fiber**

Apple Salad

This is a crunchy fall salad that is full of contrasting flavors of savory, spicy, and sweet that will definitely awaken your taste buds.

Serves 4

Ingredients:

- 3 Granny Smith apples, peel and cube
- 1 cup of low fat plain yogurt
- 1/3 cup of blue cheese crumbles
- 1/3 cup of pistachios
- ¼ teaspoon of cayenne pepper
- A squeeze of lemon juice
- ½ teaspoon of blackpepper

Directions:

1. Mix together the yogurt, cayenne pepper, black pepper, and lemon juice. Toss in the apples and gently mix until well-combined. Chill until serving time.
2. To serve, add in the pistachio and blue cheese into the salad and mix well. Serve immediately.

Nutrition Info per Serving: **200 Calories, 8.5g Total Fat, 25g Carbohydrates, 8.5g Protein and 4g Fiber**

Apple Yogurt Coleslaw

This salad has a little bit of everything nutrient-wise.

Serves 4

Ingredients:

- 1 medium Granny Smith apple, chop
- 4 cups of green cabbage, slice thinly
- 1 cup of low fat plain yogurt
- ½ cup of carrot, shredded
- 1 tablespoon of lemon juice
- 1 teaspoon of sugar
- ¼ teaspoon of salt
- ½ teaspoon of celery seeds
- A pinch of pepper

Directions:

1. Combine the carrots, apple, and cabbage in a bowl.

2.   In a separate bowl, combine the yogurt, lemon juice, sugar, salt, celery seeds, and pepper. Pour the mixture over the salad and mix well until well-coated.

3.   Chill for 8 hours. Serve immediately.

Nutrition Info per Serving: **100 Calories, 1g Total Fat, 19g Carbohydrates, 4g Protein and 4g Fiber**

Apricot Chicken Pasta Salad

This salad is perfect for the apricot season.

Serves 4

Ingredients:

For the dressing

- 2 tablespoons of white wine vinegar
- 2 apricots, quartered
- 1 tablespoon of sugar
- ¼ teaspoon of salt
- 1 tablespoon of finely chopped fresh basil
- 3 tablespoons of olive oil

For the salad

- 6 fresh apricots, quartered

- ¼ lb of fusilli pasta
- 2 skinless and boneless chicken breasts
- 2 cups of low sodium chicken broth
- 2 small zucchini, trim ends and cut to make thin strips
- 1 red bell pepper, cut to make thin strips
- 1 tablespoon of chopped fresh basil

Directions:

1. Add the sugar, salt, white wine vinegar, and apricots in a blender and process until smooth.

2. While the blender is turned on, slowly drizzle in the olive oil and mix until smooth and thick. Stir in the basil. Set aside until needed.

3. Add the chicken broth in a saucepan and bring to boil. Reduce the temperature and add in the chicken breasts. Simmer for 6 minutes.

4. Remove the chicken from the saucepan. Once cool enough to handle, shred the chicken to make bite size pieces.

5. Cook the pasta as the package directs. Let cool then combine with the basil, red pepper, zucchini, apricots, and chicken in a salad bowl. Add in the dressing and toss lightly until well-coated.

Nutrition Info per Serving: **360 Calories, 15g Total Fat, 36g Carbohydrates, 11g Protein and 4g Fiber**

Avocado Egg Salad

This creamy and yummy salad is quick to make and can be taken on-the-go.

Serves 6

Ingredients:

- 4 hard-boiled egg whites, chop
- 4 large hard-boiled eggs, chop, separate white and yolk
- 1 tablespoon of light mayonnaise
- 1 medium avocado, cut to make ½-inch pieces
- ½ tablespoon of finely chopped chives
- 1 tablespoon of fat-free plain yogurt
- ½ teaspoon of salt
- 2 teaspoons of red wine vinegar
- ¼ teaspoon of freshly ground pepper

Directions:

1. Mix together all of the ingredients in a salad bowl and toss gently until well-combined.

Nutrition Info per Serving: **114 Calories, 8g Total Fat, 4g Carbohydrates, 8g Protein and 1g Fiber**

Fall Spinach Salad

This quick fall salad is full of Vitamin A and fiber.

Serves 4

Ingredients:

- 1/8 teaspoon of salt
- 1 tablespoon of honey
- 1 tablespoon of olive oil
- 1 ¼ lbs of butternut squash, peel and dice to make ¾-inch pieces

For the vinaigrette

- 1 ½ tablespoons of white balsamic vinegar
- 1 ½ tablespoons of olive oil
- ½ tablespoon of minced shallots
- 1 tablespoon of honey
- 2 teaspoons of Dijon mustard

For the salad

- ¼ cup of raw and hulled pumpkin seeds

- 5 oz baby spinach, wash and spin dry
- ¼ cup of reduced fat crumbled gorgonzola
- 3 tablespoons of dried cherries

Directions:

1. Turn on the oven and set to 400F.

2. Season the butternut squash with 1/8 teaspoon of salt, 1 tablespoon of honey, and 1 tablespoon of olive oil. Once well-coated, place the butternut squash on a baking sheet and roast for 25 minutes. Let cool while preparing the rest of the salad.

3. Whisk together all the ingredients for the vinaigrette and toss together all the salad ingredients. Place the salad on a bowl and top with the roasted butternut squash. Drizzle the dressing over the salad and serve.

Nutrition Info per Serving: **240 Calories, 11g Total Fat, 35g Carbohydrates, 5g Protein and 8g Fiber**

Summer Barley Salad

Enjoy this yummy mixture of fruits and vegetables. It's definitely a crowd-pleaser so you'll want to bring this to potlucks.

Serves 10

Ingredients:

- 3 cups of water
- 1 cup of dry barley
- 1 cup of fresh blueberries
- ¼ cup of dried cranberries
- ½ cup of red bell pepper, chop
- 1 cup of sweet snap peas
- ½ cup of green onions, slice thinly
- 2 cups of apples, chop
- 3 tablespoons of vegetable oil
- 1 tablespoon of vinegar
- ¼ cup of lemon juice

Directions:

1. Add the water and barley in a saucepan then bring to boil. Set the temperature to low and cover the saucepan with a lid. Cook for 45 minutes.

2.   Rinse the barley in cold water. Drain and add the remaining ingredients. Toss until well-combined. Serve immediately.

Nutrition Info per Serving: **150 Calories, 5g Total Fat, 26g Carbohydrates, 3g Protein and 5g Fiber**

Colorful Corn and Barley Salad

This high-fiber colorful salad goes great with fish or chicken.

Serves 12

Ingredients:

- 15 oz of kidney beans, drain
- 2 cups of cooked pearl barley
- 1 large red bell pepper, seeded and chop finely
- 1 cup of corn
- ¼ cup of sliced green onion
- ½ cup of sliced celery
- ¼ cup of fresh lemon juice
- 1 clove of garlic, chop finely
- 1/8 teaspoon of salt
- 2 tablespoons of vegetable oil

- Fresh cilantro
- ¼ teaspoon of pepper

Directions:

1.   Add the water and barley in a saucepan then bring to boil. Set the temperature to low and cover the saucepan with a lid. Cook for 45 minutes.

2.   Rinse the barley in cold water. Drain and add the remaining ingredients except for the cilantro. Cover and refrigerate overnight. Top with fresh cilantro before serving.

Nutrition Info per Serving: **110 Calories, 3g Total Fat, 19g Carbohydrates, 4g Protein and 5g Fiber**

Corn and Black Bean Salsa Salad

With its simple but refreshing flavors, this truly is the best salad for grilling season.

Serves 8

Ingredients:

For the dressing

- ¼ cup of fresh lime juice
- 1/3 cup of olive oil
- ½ teaspoon of ground cumin
- 1 clove of garlic, mince
- ½ teaspoon of ground coriander

For the salad

- 2 cups of corn kernels
- 2 cups of cooked black beans
- ¾ cup of orange bell pepper, remove the seeds then chop
- ¾ cup of red bell pepper, remove the seeds then chop
- ¾ cup of sweet red onion, chop finely
- 2 small jalapcno chilies, remove the seeds then mince
- ½ cup of fresh cilantro, chop finely
- 1 large ripe tomato, chop

Directions:

1. Make the dressing by whisking together the coriander, cumin, garlic, lime juice, and olive oil in a small bowl until well-combined. Set aside for half an hour to let the flavors blend together.

2. To make the salad, combine the onion, jalapenos, bell peppers, corn, and black beans in a

salad bowl. Pour the dressing over the mixture and toss until well-coated. Add in the chopped tomatoes and toss again.

3. Cover the salad with cling wrap and chill for a couple of hours to let the flavors meld together. Toss in the parsley and cilantro before serving.

Nutrition Info per Serving: **190 Calories, 9.5g Total Fat, 23g Carbohydrates, 6g Protein and 6g Fiber**

Conclusion

I hope this book helped you understand the basic concept of the DASH diet and how it can help you prevent numerous health risks by providing you with healthier food options. Also, I hope you have enjoyed the recipes as much as we did.

The next step is to use what you have learned to develop new habits to become healthier and to create new recipes you can share with the DASH diet community.

Lastly, if you enjoyed reading the book, could you please take time to share your views with us by posting a review on Amazon? Having a positive review from you helps the book reach many more people, so we can continue to reach those who can benefit from the information shared within the book. It'd be highly appreciated!

Thanks again for purchasing this book and good luck with your journey to better health!

Part II

DASH Diet

The Ultimate DASH Diet Guide to Lose Weight, Lower Blood Pressure, and Stop Hypertension Fast

Introduction

Hypertension is one of the world's most notorious silent killers. It develops insidiously, without any warning signs. A person may enjoy normal daily activities only to suddenly drop to floor, unconscious. Subsequent medical tests would reveal hypertension. However, at that point, the condition would have wreaked havoc and cause damage to numerous tissues.

You can stop hypertension by following a healthy diet. DASH or Dietary Approaches to Stop Hypertension is an eating plan designed to naturally and effectively manage hypertension. Aside from that, DASH promotes other benefits, including weight loss.

Find out more about these things and more by reading this book.

DASH Diet is one diet plan that'll surely help you become healthier, with less risk of acquiring numerous scary diseases like cancer and diabetes. More than that, DASH Diet may prove to be the only thing you need to achieve a slimmer body without having to spend hours sweating out in the gym.

Read this book now and change your life for the better.

CHAPTER 1

What is the DASH Diet?

DASH Diet is Dietary Approaches to Stop Hypertension. Hypertension affects over 1 billion people worldwide, from all walks of like, from different age brackets. Hypertension is not only seen in the elderly. Even young, healthy young adults are also affected. Cases of young children and teenagers with hypertension are also not uncommon.

For years, experts have tried to understand what causes hypertension and the reason why some people cannot seem to recover from the condition. One of the theories was diet. Scientists believed that certain food components could push the body to maintain higher blood pressure. With that, the research community focused on diet, namely, determining what foods promote hypertension, and of course, what foods can prevent it from occurring or manage the condition.

Basics of DASH Diet

DASH Diet is originally intended for people with or at risk of developing hypertension. This was part of treatment and prevention of high blood pressure and for heart diseases.

The focus of the diet is on healthier food choices. It recommended eating more whole grains, vegetables, lean meats and fruits.

Updated version of the diet also included restrictions on sodium intake.

This diet was created based on scientific research results. Researchers observed that people who followed a more plant-based diet had less risk for hypertension. For instance, there are fewer vegetarians and vegans who suffer from hypertension than people with diets mainly consisting of meat.

Researchers noted that large amounts of certain nutrients might play an important role. These nutrients are found more in grains, vegetables, lean meats and fruits. It was also noted that plant-based diets had less added sugars, which might also help prevent the disease.

Plant-based diets also have less sodium. In the DASH Diet, sodium intake should not exceed 2,300 mg per day or no more than 1 teaspoon. For those who needed sodium restriction (i.e., suffering or at high risk for cardiovascular disorders like congestive heart failure), sodium intake should not exceed 1,500 mg per day or no more than ¾ teaspoon.

What is DASH Diet?

Experts found that hypertension can be improved by making simple changes in diet. According to the first research on the effectiveness of DASH Diet, even a person with a 3,000 mg sodium intake per day and is hypertensive will experience a large reduction in blood pressure. Research was sponsored by the US

National Institute for Health. This was part of the efforts to deal with hypertension without taking medications.

Recent researches in hypertension found that sodium also plays an important role in how the condition develops. Hence, DASH Diet evolved into including sodium reduction in its diet plan. For instance, simply lowering sodium intake by 6 grams/day will already bring down blood pressure by as much as 7/4 mmHg in hypertensive patients.

That effect lasts for days and weeks. Medications may lower blood pressure by as much or even greater but only for a few hours. Blood pressure will be further reduced by the cumulative effect of the various compounds in the healthy foods in the DASH Diet.

Over the years, DASH Diet research revealed more benefits. This diet plan alone can significantly reduce the risks for serious diseases affecting the kidneys, liver and heart. It can reduce the development of diabetes, heart failure, stroke, and even cancer.

Improved DASH Diet

Further research found that DASH Diet can still be improved. Results from other nutritional research found that refined foods are bad for health. Improvements were made and DASH Diet now is less on starchy food sand refined grains.

Research continued and more improvements were made. Cutting back on "empty carbs" promoted better results and greater decline in BP. This improvement made DASH Diet more weight-loss friendly. Furthermore, DASH is now more focused on adding heart-healthy fats and more proteins.

Other benefits of DASH

DASH is more than just a natural anti-hypertensive lifestyle. It promotes other benefits, such as:

- Weight loss

- Lower cancer risk, such as reduced risk for breast and colorectal cancer

- Reduced risk for heart diseases, as shown in one recent review wherein women on DASH experienced 20% less risk for heart diseases and 29% less risk for strokes.

- Reduced risk for diabetes, mainly from less intake of sugary and processed foods, as well as the consequent weight loss. Food and lifestyle in DASH also promotes reduced insulin resistance of the tissues.

- Reduced risk for metabolic syndrome, as shown in studies, which can be as much as an 81% risk reduction

- Overall reduced risk for numerous diseases such as PCOS and post-menopausal weight gain. This is due to the healthier diet and the removal of disease-promoting artificial food ingredients in most processed foods.

CHAPTER 2

Why was the DASH Diet Created?

The DASH Diet plan was originally created as a natural way to address hypertension. Log-term use of anti-hypertensives can result in some negative side effects. There is also the risk that the body learns to depend on these drugs to regulate blood pressure. Long term use of medications can also cause some damage to the kidneys and the liver.

Besides, the BP-lowering effects of these anti-hypertensive drugs are temporary. A patient would have to take these regularly every day to manage hypertension.

Hence, the DASH Diet was created.

Dietary Approaches to Stop Hypertension soon became an integral part of hypertension management. The best part about this plan is that the effects go beyond lowering BP. It is actually a lifestyle that everyone can benefit from. This diet may be initially developed for hypertension but it can be enjoyed by everyone. Both healthy people and individuals suffering from any disease can benefit from this diet/lifestyle.

Who is DASH Diet for?

Research showed that this diet is effective in reducing blood pressure down to normal ranges in both healthy and hypertensive people. Scientific evidence showed that this diet alone can lower

BP even if the person does not restrict salt (sodium) intake or lose weight.

If DASH Diet is done with sodium restriction, BP goes down even further. Results proved that sodium restriction and DASH produced the greatest reductions in BP.

This combination resulted in an average of 11 points reduction in BP in those suffering from hypertension. Normal healthy people experienced a 3-point reduction in their BP levels.

A Short Look at Hypertension

The force of blood that flows through the blood vessels is called blood pressure. This is measured using 2 parameters- the systolic and the diastolic.

Systolic blood pressure is the pressure exerted on the blood vessels when the heart contracts. Diastolic pressure is pressure exerted on the blood vessels when the heart is relaxed.

Normal blood pressure ranges from 100/60 to 120/80. The upper value is systolic blood pressure. The lower value is diastolic blood pressure.

High blood pressure is when the readings are above 140/90.

High blood pressure of hypertension is a serious health issue. It is widely considered as the silent killer. There are no obvious signs that someone is suffering from this condition. People think they are unaffected only to fall seriously ill at a moment's notice. Most often, symptoms appear when the person already has alarmingly high blood pressure and damage to organs have been great.

Some of the symptoms a person with extremely high blood pressure are:

- Severe headache
- Vision problems
- Fatigue or confusion
- Pounding in your chest, neck, or ears
- Chest pain
- Irregular heartbeat
- Difficulty breathing
- Blood in the urine

Experts estimate that more people have hypertension than is actually diagnosed because of the absence of early symptoms. This is why the DASH Diet and adopting a healthy lifestyle is recommended for everyone. This is not a diet only for those already diagnosed for hypertension.

CHAPTER 3

Characteristics of the DASH Diet

This diet puts more focus on healthy plant-based food choices. Fiber intake is highly encouraged. Minerals and vitamins are obtained from healthy plant sources. Proteins are from both plant sources and lean animal sources. These are taken in moderation. Healthy fats are also included. These are taken in moderate quantities. Sodium intake is controlled.

Meals are mostly vegetables and fruits, along with whole grains. Meats and fats are taken in moderation. Meats should be lean, with as much visible fat and all the skin removed prior to cooking. Poultry and fish are also included as sources of both healthy proteins and fats. Dairy is included, as long as it is non-fat or low fat.

Sodium intake in the DASH Diet follows the US guidelines for salt intake. Some people might need to reduce their salt intake further due to certain heath conditions. For instance, people suffering from congestive heart failure might have to severely limit their salt intake. People with extremely high blood pressures might also have to reduce their sodium intake lower than the US guidelines. Some people, on the other hand, might not need such as restrictions. Examples are those on medications, activities and health conditions that require them to take more sodium for better electrolyte balance.

DASH Diet is considered by some people as the American version of the healthy Mediterranean diet. These two diets share a lot of similarities. Both focus more on plant foods, with low to moderate intake of animal and animal-based foods. Dairy is also included but in low to moderate quantities. Meals are also rich in nuts and seeds, as well as legumes and beans. Whole grain also takes up a good percentage of each meal.

The DASH Diet is originally for lowering BP. It wasn't really a weight loss plan. It is a flexible diet that allowed followers to choose from a large variety of foods. There is no strict food list. The most basic guideline was to eat more fiber from whole grains, fruits and vegetables.

Years of research and feedback from those who followed the diet led to a few modifications. These modifications were based on results of nutritional studies. For instance, research found that refined sugar and grains are unhealthy. Foods that contain these ingredients are no longer recommended under DASH Diet. There is now emphasis on whole grains. Now, DASH Diet has various versions for specific health and nutrition needs.

Recommendations of the DASH Diet Plan

The plan gives suggested servings on important food groups. Some give recommendations for daily intake while others are for weekly intake. Some foods need to be eaten daily to provide the necessary daily nutrient needs.

The prevailing DASH Diet guidelines on servings are based on a 2,000 calorie per day diet allocation.

Food Group	Daily Servings
Grains	6–8
Fruit	4–5
Vegetables	4–5
Meats, poultry, and fish	6 or less
Fats and oils	2–3
Low-fat or fat-free dairy products	2–3
Sodium	2,300 mg*

*For sodium intake, work with a doctor especially when other diseases, medications or risk factors are present. Sodium may need to be further restricted to 1, 500 mg for those with higher risk for conditions such as congestive heart failure.

Some food groups are not necessarily needed to be taken every single day. Weekly serving allocations are still just as important for good health and lower BP.

Food Group	Weekly Servings
Sweets	5 or less
Nuts, seeds, dry beans, and peas	4–5

CHAPTER 4

DASH Diet Food Groups

DASH Diet promotes the daily intake of specific food groups. All these food groups are highly recommended to be consumed daily, at certain recommended servings. The recommended servings from each food group are carefully designed to fit into a 2,000 calorie-per-day diet.

Grains

This is a vital food group for DASH Diet for many reasons. Grains are the diet's major source of fiber and energy.

Fiber helps in lowering blood pressure levels in many ways. It can help in lowering cholesterol levels in the blood. It can absorb toxins and excess substances, bringing it out of the body through your bowel movement.

Fiber also helps the body absorb more nutrients from food. By adding grains, the body optimizes digestion and absorption of food. Benefits from these nutrients can be optimized as well.

Servings per day: 6 to 8

Grain servings may include pasta, cereal, bread and rice. Stay away from refined grains. Choose whole grains instead. Whole grains contain more nutrients and fiber compared to refined grains. Refined processing destroys most of the fiber, where most of the nutrients are attached to.

Make better food choices through substitutions. Instead of eating white rice, eat brown rice instead. Choose whole grain breads and whole wheat pasta instead of regular pasta and white breads.

Vegetables

Fresh vegetables are rich in minerals and vitamins. Minerals like potassium and magnesium help in normal functioning of the cardiovascular system. Magnesium, for instance, helps with normal rhythm and strength of heart contractions. This can contribute to better regulation of BP. Potassium helps regulate the volume of blood. How much blood flowing through the blood vessels plays an important role in BP regulation.

DASH Diet incorporates vegetables as a huge percentage of a meal, as opposed to being merely side dishes or garnishes. It is recommended that you add a good helping of vegetables to whole wheat pasta dishes or over steamed browned rice. Mix in with whole wheat noodles for a hearty main meal.

Both fresh and frozen vegetables can be used for different recipes. Fresh and in season are always best. At this period, the minerals and vitamin contents are at the peak, not to mention the excellent flavor.

For frozen vegetables, check that there are no added sodium. Some vegetables have added salt to serve as natural preservative. Check labels and choose frozen vegetables with less or no added salt.

Servings per day: 4 to 5

Vegetable servings include a variety of choices. There are leafy green vegetables like lettuce, cabbage, kale, spinach and arugula. There are the several varieties of squashes, peppers, radishes and zucchini. There are carrots, peas and eggplants. There are just so many choices to keep meals interesting and flavorful.

Daily recommended serving is 4-5. It will be easier to get these much if vegetables are treated as part of the main dish rather than as toppings or side dishes. Meat servings in a recipe may be halved and replaced with more vegetables to increase how much vegetables you eat every day.

Fruits

This is another important food group. Frits contain minerals and vitamins that improve health. Most of these act as antioxidants. Toxins may contribute to high blood pressure as it causes damage to the tissues and lining of the blood vessels. Toxins and free radicals may also cause imbalances that contribute to higher BP.

Most fruits are also low in fat. Some, like coconut, contain fat but of the good kind. Monounsaturated fat in coconut is even good for the heart and blood vessels. It may also lower BP and reduce risk for heart diseases.

There are many ways to get fruits into the daily diet. Fruits are healthy snacks. Have some cut-up fruits in small containers as ready-to-eat snacks. These are also healthier dessert options to round up a healthy, hearty DASH meal. You may also add a small dollop of healthy low fat yogurt to make a more delicious treat.

Eat fruits with the peel, if possible. Most of the antioxidants and fiber are found in the peel. The texture and tartness of the peel help create a wonderful contrasting flavor to the sweetness of the fruit's flesh.

Fruits are healthy. However, some fruits may interact with certain medications so take caution. For instance, grapefruit may interact with some antidepressant drugs. Other citrus fruits and juices may interact as well so consult a health care provider.

Servings per day: 4 to 5

DASH Diet recommends eating 4 to 5 servings of fruits per day. Fresh fruits are best but you may also eat canned or frozen fruits. Check the label to see there are no added sugars. Also check for any added sodium in these products.

Dairy

These are excellent sources of calcium, proteins and vitamin D. Proteins help promote tissue repair and maintenance. This can help in reducing inflammation due to tissue injuries. Reduced inflammation contributes to reduced BP levels.

Calcium is an important nutrient in muscle function. This plays a role in regulating the contraction of muscles, including the muscles of the heart, tissue muscles and muscles that line the blood vessels. A healthy amount of calcium helps the heart and blood vessels to contract and dilate normally. This is a huge step towards lowering blood pressure. Tissues that are also functioning well means that there is less resistance for blood flow, leading to reduced BP.

However, it is important to be choosy when it comes to dairy. Choose dairy low in fat or fat-free. Otherwise, dairy products become major fat sources in the diet.

The type of fat that dairy products contain is not always the healthy type. Most of these fats are saturated fats. This type of fat is huge contributor to the development of cardiovascular diseases, including hypertension. Do note that not all saturated fats are bad. These are still used by the body. However, taking too much can cause some health problems. Taking full fat dairy products each day results to a large intake of saturated fats that may not prove healthy for the body.

To get the other nutrients in dairy but not the fats, choose fat-free or low-fat versions.

Some people may have lactose intolerance. This should not hinder taking dairy products every day. There are lactose-free versions available to reduce symptoms of lactose intolerance. Another option is to take enzyme lactase. This product is available over-the-counter, which means prescription is not needed when purchasing. This can help reduce symptoms of lactose intolerance when eating dairy products.

Intake of dairy every day isn't that difficult. Aside from drinking a glass of milk every day, dairy can be added to various dishes. These can even be healthier alternatives to sodium-rich commercial dressings. For instance, instead of fatty Caesar salad dressing from the store, mix herbs and spices with some low-fat yogurt. Instead of high sodium, high fat commercially bottled pasta sauce, cook warm white sauce with 1% milk. Make soups creamier by adding some skim milk. add a splash of low fat milk to coffee, tea, smoothies and shakes. Top a bowl of fruit with frozen yogurt for a delicious dessert or refreshing snack. Add skim milk, low-fat milk, 1% milk or yogurt to muesli or whole grain breakfast cereals. Top vegetable omelet with fat-free, low sodium cheese for a heartier breakfast. The options are endless.

Servings per day: 2 to 3

The recommended daily intake of dairy is 2 to 3 servings. There are many choices, not just milk. There are skim milk and yogurt. Milk comes in numerous low fat versions such as 1% milk. There are numerous types of cheeses. Do be careful with cheese choices. Some are high in sodium and fats. Best to avoid regular cheese, especially processed cheese. Even some fat-free cheeses may contain too much sodium so always check the label.

Fish, poultry or lean meats

These are rich sources of proteins. These are also good sources of B vitamins, zinc and iron. Organ meats, for instance, are rich in iron that helps with proper blood cell production. This contributes to the regulation of normal BP.

Healthy fats can also be obtained from fishes. Cold water fishes such as salmon and cod are rich in omacids.

Servings per day: less than 6 servings

Lean varieties are highly advised. Aim to get less than 6 servings per day. DASH Diet actually suggests cutting back meat intake and make room for more vegetables.

Remove all visible fats from the meats. This is highly recommended when eating poultry, beef and pork. Remove the skin, too. In poultry, most of the fat is found in the skin. Remove it all.

Fats from fishes are healthier. These are omega-3 fatty acids that protect the body from cardiovascular diseases. It also reduces inflammation that contributes to the development of hypertension. Some fishes also contain monounsaturated fats. This is another type of healthy fat that can help promote better health and lower BP.

Cooking the meats is also important. Avoid dishes and cooking styles that call for additional fats. Avoid sautéing, deep frying, etc. Avoid adding high sodium ingredients, too.

Healthy cooking options include:

- Broiling
- Steaming
- Baking
- Grilling
- Roasting

Nuts, legumes and seeds

Almonds, Brazil nuts, pumpkin seeds, sunflower seeds, chia seeds, lentils, peas, and lots of different types of beans are all included in the DASH Diet. These are good plant sources of proteins. These ae also rich in potassium and magnesium, too. Phytochemicals and fiber are also abundant in these foods. Phytochemicals may help protect the body from different cardiovascular diseases and certain cancers.

Some people stay away from nuts because of the fat contents. Nuts do contain fats but the healthy kind -- omega-3 fats and monounsaturated fats.

Nuts and seeds make healthy snacks. A handful is enough, though so careful not to eat too much. Get the dry roasted ones, not deep fried.

Seeds and nuts are also perfect to add in various DASH dishes. These can be crunchy toppings to salads. You can also encrust lean meats in seeds or crushed nuts for some interesting texture and flavor. Chia seeds can be added to numerous salads, soups and meat dishes. These can be added to smoothies as well for some crunch. Almonds can be added to smoothies to make it creamier. Cereals with an assortment of seeds and nuts, with a few fruit slices make a delicious, filling, heart-healthy DASH meal.

There is an endless list of ways to eat more beans. These can be made into soups, chilies, baked beans, steamed, boiled, etc.

Soy beans made into tofu and tempeh are also good to add. These can be healthier substitutes for meats. These have a meaty, earthy flavor that can be added to numerous dishes. Soy beans contain all the essential amino acids that the body needs.

Servings per week: 4 to 5

Note that DASH Diet recommends this food group with 4-5 servings per **week**, not per day. The calories will add up. It is easy to finish a large bag of nuts in one sitting. That would pack in a substantial amount of calories.

Fats and Oils

Fats and oils are important nutrients. Some people ask this question:

Don't fats and oils contribute to cardiovascular diseases?

Yes and no.

It depends on the type of fats and how much is eaten regularly.

First off, too much saturated fat from bad sources is bad for health. In controlled amounts and from healthy sources, saturated fats are good for health.

Omega-3 fatty acid is a good type of fat. It has numerous benefits that can help reduce BP. It reduces inflammation, fights free radicals and promotes better blood flow.

Inflammation gets in the way of proper blood flow. It makes the lumen (space in the middle of the blood vessel where blood flows through

Servings per day: 2 to 3

Healthy fats is key and in moderation. DASH Diet promotes fat intake to be no more than 30% of daily calorie intake. Emphasis is on healthy fats such as monounsaturated fats. This type of fat shows protective action on the cardiovascular system against diseases such as plaque formation along the blood vessels and inflammation.

When eating fats, limit intake of saturated fats. You do not have to totally cut out this fat from the diet. It is useful but only in controlled amounts. Keep intake of saturated fats to no more than 6% of total daily calorie intake. Saturated fats are found in foods like:

- Whole milk
- Cheese
- Meat
- Eggs
- Cream
- Butter
- Food made with coconut and palm oils
- Foods made with solid shortening
- Foods made with lard

Trans-fats must be avoided. Numerous researches showed that trans -fat is unusable in the body. Furthermore, trans fats are strongly linked to the development of cardiovascular diseases, obesity and cancer. This unhealthy, artificial form of fat can be found in processed foods such as crackers, fried foods and baked goods.

Sweets

Sweets may still be enjoyed by those on the DASH Diet. However, this must be in controlled portions. Healthy swaps may also help enjoy those sweet treats without packing in calories.

Refined sugars should be avoided. These are high in calories but empty in nutrition. Avoid all foods that contain refined sugar such as chips and processed sweets.

Artificial sweeteners may be used but sensibly. Even this can turn unhealthy is used in excess. Aspartame and sucralose are common artificial sweeteners that can be used. Aspartame is marketed as Equal and NutraSweet. Sucralose is marketed as Splenda.

Diet cola can be swapped for regular cola. However, it is better to drink healthier beverages such as plain water and low fat milk.

*Servings per **week**: 5 or fewer*

DASH Diet allows for sweets, in controlled portions. Choose low-fat or fat-free versions. Examples are:

- Low fat cookies
- Graham crackers
- Jelly beans
- Fruit ices
- Sorbets
- Hard candy

Alcohol, Caffeine

These two are still allowed but in limited amounts. Drinking too much caffeine and alcohol can increase BP levels.

DASH Diet follows the Dietary Guidelines for Americans regarding alcohol consumption. Men should take care not to drink alcohol drinks exceeding 2 drinks per day. Women should not exceed 1 drink per day.

With caffeine, there is no clear guideline. The exact effect of caffeine on BP is still not defined. Some people experience rise in BP after consuming certain amounts of caffeine. Some people don't.

What is clear is that caffeine can raise BP temporarily, at the least. The rise might be sustained for a few hours. There is no definite guideline yet on what caffeine levels create what range of BP increase. It is mainly on individual responses. Some people experience a huge rise in BP after consuming a cup of espresso. Some people may only experience a small increase with that same amount of caffeine.

Regulating caffeine is mainly based on working closely with a doctor. If a person feels that caffeine intake may affect their BP levels, talk to a doctor for further assessment and possible steps to take.

CHAPTER 5

Portion Control and Serving Sizes

Portion control is a vital component in DASH Diet. You can't expect to lower your BP while overindulging on cheese or salmon. You can't expect to meet your weight loss goals while piling up on almonds. Good health won't result from eating too much fruits or eating one group of vegetables only. All the benefits of DASH Diet can only be achieved by eating well-balanced meals.

Balance is achieved by ensuring that certain food groups are included at each meal. These food groups are whole grains, meats (or poultry, seafood), vegetables, fruits, oils, fats and dairy.

DASH Diet Servings Per Food Group

As discussed in detail from the previous chapter, here is a summary of the recommended servings for various food groups:

- Grains: 7-8 daily servings

- Fruits: 4-5 daily servings

- Vegetables: 4-5 daily servings

- Fish, meat, and poultry: 2 or less daily servings

- Dairy products, fat-free or low-fat: 2-3 daily servings

- Fats, oils: 2-3 daily servings

- Seeds, nuts, and dry beans: 4-5 servings per week

- Sweets: try to limit to less than 5 servings per week

How much is 1 serving?

DASH Diet recommends 6-8 servings of whole grains each day. One serving typically looks like any of these:

- 1 ounce of dry cereal

- ½ cup of cooked pasta, rice or cereal

- 1 slice of whole wheat bread

One serving of vegetables looks like any of these:

- ½ cup of cooked or raw sliced vegetables

- 1 cup of raw green leafy vegetables

A serving of fruits may be any of the following:

- One medium-sized fruit

- ½ cup of cut-up frozen, canned or fresh fruits

- 4 ounces of fruit juice

A serving of dairy looks like any of these:

- 1 cup of low fat yogurt

- 1 cup of 1% milk

- 1 cup of skim milk

- 1 ½ ounces of part-skim cheese

- 8 ounces of milk

A serving of seeds, nuts and legumes looks like any of these:

- 2 tablespoons of seeds

- ½ cup of cooked peas or beans

- 1/3 cup of nuts

One serving of fat looks like any of these:

- 1 tablespoon of mayonnaise

- 2 tablespoons of salad dressings

- 1 teaspoon of soft margarine

- 1 teaspoon of olive oil (or any other oil)

One serving of sweets look like any of these:

- 1 tablespoon of sugar, jam or jelly

- 1 cup of lemonade

- ½ cup of sorbet

One serving of meats, fish & poultry looks like any of these:

- 3 ounces tofu

- 3 ounces cooked meat

Servings per day

In the previous chapter, the serving recommendations were based on a 2,000 calorie diet. This is what most people recommend and follow when adopting the DASH Diet plan.

Some people can follow the 1,500 calorie per if trying to lose weight. Some people may need higher calorie intakes for their individual health goals (e.g., those who need to beef up, etc.).

CHAPTER 6

DASH Diet Food List

DASH Diet is heavy on fruits, grains and vegetables. For DASH for Hypertension, dairy, lean meats, poultry and fish are also included. Sweets are also allowed.

To get a better idea on what foods are recommended by DASH Diet plan, here's a comprehensive list.

Fruits

- Apples

- Berries

- Bananas

- Grapes

- Raisins

- Lime

- Lemon

- Pineapples

- Pear

Vegetables

- Artichokes

- Bell peppers

- Broccoli

- Carrots

- Cabbage

- Cauliflower

- Green beans

- Corn

- Lettuce

- Mushrooms

- Onions

- Potatoes

- Squash

- Sprouts

Meats, Seafood

- Chicken

- Beef

- Eggs

- Salmon

- Turkey

- Shrimp

Breads, Grains

- Brown rice

- Whole grain cereal

- Barley

- Some oats

- Whole wheat bread

- Whole wheat pasta

- Whole wheat tortillas

- Wild rice

Nuts, Seeds

- Peanuts

- Almonds

- Pecans

- Cashews

- Walnuts

- Pumpkin seeds

Dairy

- Cottage cheese

- Fat-free yogurt

- Reduced-fat cheese

- Fat-free milk

- Sour cream

- Margarine

CHAPTER 7

The DASH Diet and Weight Loss

DASH Diet was originally created for hypertensive patients. It is a healthy dietary plan and its benefits extend beyond lowering BP. It can also be used as an effective, sustainable diet plan for weight loss. Besides, a hypertensive person is most likely advised to lose weight. Excess body weight is one of the leading risk factors for hypertension.

Following DASH Diet is actually a brilliant way to stay healthy and achieve a slimmer body. DASH Diet can also promote weight loss. When excess weight is removed, hypertension can be further reduced. It's a cycle that promotes greater benefits as it progresses.

How DASH Diet can lead to weight loss

DASH Diet recommends eating more whole grains, vegetables and fruits. These are at the core of majority of the weight loss diet plans. These are in fiber and low in calories. To lose weight, a person must reduce calorie intake. This would usually mean eating less frequently and with fewer servings. Grains, vegetables and fruits allow a person to eat more servings and more often without loading up on calories.

Fiber also helps a person to feel full sooner into a meal. This greatly helps in controlling portion sizes. Fiber also helps to feel full longer. This helps to reduce the frequency of eating.

Grains, vegetables and fruits are also rich in micronutrients such as vitamins and minerals. These help in improving tissue functions for improved nutrient absorption and use. This helps in fast-tracking weight loss and sustaining it.

See, poor tissue nutrition contributes to weight gain. If the cells are not absorbing enough nutrients, hunger signals will be created. You will be eating more and absorbing less. Unabsorbed nutrients may be converted into fats that contribute to weight gain and obesity.

The other healthy choices also help in losing weight. For instance, DASH Diet recommends lean meats and healthier animal meats like poultry and fish. These choices are other major factors in weight loss plans.

DASH Diet also promotes specific servings for each food group. This helps in regulating portion sizes and further controlling calorie intake. This, again, is a major factor when trying to lose weight.

DASH Diet is also about healthy living. It promotes not just healthy diet but regular exercise as well. In weight loss, diet plays a major role, exercise having less impact on weight loss. However, regular exercise can help in speeding up metabolism. It also contributes to burning excess fats and mobilizing stored fats to be converted into usable energy.

CHAPTER 8

Tips to Make the Switch to DASH Diet Eating

For some people, making a switch to the DASH Diet may be quite a challenge. This diet is not a temporary eating plan. For DASH Diet to work and effectively lower BP, this eating plan must be embraced and treated as a lifestyle. It's not something to be followed for only a few weeks or days. It has to be a lifetime eating plan.

To make the switch easier, check out these strategies.

Gradual change

Give time for the body and the mind to get accustomed to the change. For someone used to eat mostly refined grain and refined sugar products, eating mostly vegetables and whole grains can be quite challenging. Limiting fatty meats and full cream dairy may turn meals into bland-looking fares.

Besides, a person not used to eating a lot of fiber may experience discomforts with a sudden change into a fiber-rich diet. Side effects can include bloating, gas and constipation or diarrhea. Give the body time to adjust to reduce these discomforts.

As previously mentioned, DASH Diet is more a lifestyle than a temporary diet. Any benefits obtained from this diet will not be maintained if a person goes back to unhealthy eating, i.e., eating unhealthy fats, refined grains and refined sugars.

Make gradual changes.

Nobody is expected to make a complete 180-degree shift to DASH Diet in a day.

Gradually easing into the DASH life makes it easier to stick to the guidelines. It will also be easier to take DASH as a lifestyle than when rapidly shifting diets.

Try these tips in making gradual changes to shift into the DASH lifestyle:

- Mix whole grains into usual grain-based meals. For example, if you usually eat a panini for lunch, try having it with whole grain bagels. Instead of boxed cereals, try having muesli. Instead of a chocolate snack bar, try some granola bars (dipped in dark chocolate if you do not want to give up some sweet indulgence).

- To get more vegetables, try an open-face sandwich or ditch the white bread altogether. Instead of vegetables as merely toppings of side dish, try having dishes that highlight vegetables. For example, instead of steak with a side of coleslaw, try whole wheat pasta with sun-dried tomatoes, a heap of spinach and shiitake mushrooms topped with a few thin slices of steak.

- Try juicing or blending. Green juices and smoothies are excellent and convenient ways to get more servings without having to eat piles of food all day. A glass of green smoothie can already contain about 2 servings of vegetables, ½ serving of fruit, a serving of seeds and ½ serving of fat-free or low-fat dairy. Try translating that many servings into whole foods. That'll be about 2 plates of food.

• Go easy on the beans. These are high in fiber and plant proteins that take some time to get used to. start with a tablespoon or 2 of beans over rice or pasta. Do not eat an entire burrito if this is the first time to eat beans or fiber. Over-the-counter products are available to help with gas and bloating when eating lots of fiber and beans.

• Choose leaner cuts of meat. Remove any visible fats and the skin before cooking. For instance, use skinless chicken breast instead of chicken thighs with the skin on. Limit meat-based meals to 1 meal per day. Learn to enjoy other flavors and textures from vegetables, poultry and seafood as well.

• Try mushrooms. DASH Diet does not really have to be meatless. However, meat consumption should be reduced. Adding mushrooms can help give dishes some earthy, meat-like flavors. Example is shiitake mushroom.

Forgive yourself

DASH Diet may seem limiting for some but it does allow room for mistakes. It is forgiving. When you make mistakes (and this will happen even with the most disciplined dieter), forgive yourself and move on. One cheeseburger from your favorite fast-food or a hearty meal from a restaurant isn't doomsday. There is always tomorrow to make up for any slip-ups.

To reduce the recurrence of slip-ups, know the triggers. This information will help in avoiding situations that cause slip-ups and mistakes.

For example, going to a coffee shop triggers a craving for bacon sandwich on white bread. Passing by a fast-food establishment makes it impossible to resist some greasy, salty French fries. Avoid these places, then.

Situations may also trigger mistakes. A party can easily be a place for eating salty finger foods, fatty dishes and foods made with refined flours, grains and sugars. This is also one situation where it is easy to drink too much alcohol.

If you can't steer clear of these places and situations, then be prepared for it. Eating a healthy DASH meal before meeting others for a party or some get-together helps. A full stomach makes it easier to keep the resolve not to order something that isn't DASH.

Reward yourself

Keep your motivation high by rewarding yourself. Rewards do not have to be food. For example, evaluating your weekly accomplishments showed you were able to stay within the diet recommendations. Mark that as an accomplishment and treat yourself to a movie or a new hook. A spa treat is also good to relax both mind and body.

Try new flavors and textures

Meats are not the only flavorful ingredients out there. Salt is not the only ingredient that brings out flavors. Be open to try new tastes and textures.

- Use herbs- lots of it. Herbs are great in making vegetable dishes more appetizing. Meat dishes are much tastier, more flavorful and more savory than vegetable dishes. To give vegetables more character, try adding herbs. A dash of pepper and chili liven up leafy green salads. Chopped dill, basil and thyme give vegetable dishes an enticing aroma. Vegetable soups can still be savory with a few herbs like tarragon and rosemary.
- Use half salt, half herbs.

Healthier Substitutions

DASH Diet plan still allows people to enjoy their favorite meals, but now in a healthier way. Take these recommendations in making healthier meals by substituting certain ingredients. These substitutions make meals more DASH yet not sacrificing much of the flavors and textures that the palate is accustomed to.

Meats

Instead of:

Regular deli meats

Choose:

Specifically low-sodium deli meats

Better choice:

Fresh meats cooked in less oil

Beans

Instead of:

Regular canned beans, liquid drained

Choose:

Low-sodium or no-salt-added, rinsed

Better choice:

Homemade dry beans

Vegetables

Instead of:

Regular canned vegetables, liquid drained

Choose:

50% less salt version of canned vegetables, liquid drained

Better choice:

No-salt-added version of canned vegetables, drained then rinsed

Best choice:

Fresh vegetables

Bread

Instead of:

Corn bread

Canned biscuits

Choose:

English muffins

Regular bread

Better choice:

Whole wheat breads like whole wheat bagels

Whole grain breads like rye bread

Cheese

Instead of:

   Dry, aged cheeses

   Processed cheese

Blue cheese

   Romano cheese

   Parmesan

Choose:

   Natural, fresh cheese such as mozzarella, Colby-Jack, gouda, brie and cheddar

Better choice:

   Low-sodium varieties

   Swiss cheese

Mixed nuts

Instead of:

   Salted

Choose:

   Lightly salted

Better choice:

Unsalted

Seasonings

Instead of:

Salt

Garlic salt

Choose:

Garlic powder

Better choice:

Salt-free seasonings

Fresh herbs

Fresh spices

Dried or powdered herbs and spices

Popcorn

Instead of:

Commercial

Oil-popped

Better choice:

Air-popped

Peanut butter

Instead of:

Reduced-fat or light (peanut oil is healthy oil so no need to stay away from it)

Choose:

Regular

Better choice:

Very low-sodium

CHAPTER 9

Tips to Lower Your Sodium Intake

Sodium is another important factor in the DASH diet. Whether you are trying to lose weight, improve health, or lower BP, monitoring your sodium intake is important.

In the body, sodium is important in the regulation of fluids and electrolytes. It is also important in muscle contractions, including the contractions of the heart and walls of the blood vessels.

Sodium tends to attract water. If you have high sodium levels in the blood, volume of blood increases. More fluids will join circulating blood. Higher blood volume will cause the heart to contract harder. Both higher volume and stringer heart contractions contribute to higher BP levels.

When there are many fluids in the blood, nutrient absorption becomes less efficient. There will be more fluids entering and exiting the cells, but with fewer nutrients entering the cells. This can lead to poor nutrition that may contribute to weight gain. If the cells are not absorbing enough nutrients, hunger signals will be created. You will be eating more and absorbing less. Unabsorbed nutrients may be converted into fats that contribute to weight gain and obesity.

You can observe this the next time you eat a bag of chips. Notice that even if you just finished one entire large bag, you still do not feel full. Within the hour, you will feel hungry again and ready to devour one large greasy cheeseburger.

Natural foods contain sodium. These are called dietary sodium. This is not a real concern in health. What is a major concern is the added salt.

Processed foods and restaurant meals often contain lots of added sodium. Our taste buds have become accustomed to eating these foods that we have also been accustomed to large amounts of sodium. We think that foods are bland if there are no added salt in it.

Just as our taste buds have become accustomed to added sodium, our taste buds can be trained to enjoy foods without any added salts. Besides, DASH does not totally eradicate sodium from the diet. Again, sodium IS important. It contributes to the problem if taken in large amounts- more than what the body needs daily.

The body has the capacity to excrete excess sodium, just like with anything in excess. However, modern diets contain way too much sodium- much more than what the kidneys can handle. The kidneys are responsible for mixing excess sodium into the urine for excretion.

DASH Diet Salt Recommendation

DASH Diet plan recommends sodium intake to be around 2,300 mg. This is about 1 teaspoon of salt. At first glance, most people will say that can't possibly eat that much salt. However, certain foods contain large amounts of salt in disguise.

For example, a regular can of diced tomatoes can contain around 150 mg of sodium per serving. One can contains 3 ½ servings. If you eat a dish that uses an entire can, that will be 1,050 mg already. What about the inherent sodium content of the other ingredients in that dish? That's just one meal/dish for the day.

Ready-to-eat cereals,

Some variations of DASH Diet call for further sodium restriction. The intake can be further reduced to 1,500 mg.

However,

Why reduce salt intake?

Salt reduction can help save lives. In the UK, thousands of deaths related to cardiovascular problems have been prevented, according to numerous researches. For instance, a study found that reducing daily intake from 10 g to 6 g could lower blood pressure, reduce deaths from stroke by 16% and reduce deaths from coronary heart disease by 12%.

Another study found excessive salt intake accumulates and effects are seen after many years. In this study, increasing sodium intake by 6 grams every day for 30 years can lead to systolic BP increase by 9 mmHg.

A study demonstrated if salt does play a role in reducing BP. Both normotensive (normal BP) and hypertensive people were subjected to salt reduction. Daily salt intake was reduced by 6 grams per deciliter of blood. Both normotensive and hypertensive individuals experienced reduction in BP. Normotensive subjects experienced a 4/2 mmHg reduction (4 mmHg reduction in systolic BP and 2 mmHg reduction in diastolic BP). Hypertensive subjects experienced 7/4 mmHg reduction.

Reducing salt intake is also considered as the fastest way to reduce BP. Response can be seen within a few days. Lower salt intake can help the body to utilize any present sodium in the body. This also gives the body a chance to start clearing out sodium that has accumulated and excrete it through the kidneys.

Tips to reducing salt intake

Foods in the DASH Diet plan are already naturally low in sodium. Again, the key is to back on added salt.

Here are a few strategies to help in cutting back sodium intake further:

• Use flavorings and spices. Check that these are sodium-free though. Some store-bought flavorings and spices contain added salt.

• Do not add salt when cooking hot cereals, pasta or rice. These may taste bland at first but the taste buds will adjust in a few days. It's time to quit the traditional way of adding salt to water when cooking pasta. Adding some spices can help make these foods more flavorful. Examples are adding curry to rice, some basil to pasta or a dash of cinnamon to hot cereals.

• Drain and discard liquids from canned food then rinse well with water. This can remove a good amount of sodium from these foods. If possible, soak canned food in water for a few minutes to remove more salt. For example, soak canned beans for about 30 minutes to an hour before using to remove more salt.

• Check labels. Choose foods that are labeled "low in sodium", "very low sodium", "sodium-free", "reduced sodium", or "no salt added". Look for specific labels on sodium contents. Some products with labels indicating lower sodium contents may prove to be still high in salt.

In addition, low fat is not always low in sodium. Even some healthy foods may be high in sodium, such as turkey slices from the deli. Check for any added salt by looking at labels and/or asking how the food was made (ask specifically for any added salt).

• Start slow. One of the main reasons why people find it difficult to stick to DASH Diet is blandness. Food will taste bland if the palate was used to high sodium flavors. Start by cutting back salt use gradually until the target sodium intake level is reached. This strategy helps the taste buds to adjust and food will no longer taste bland.

• Start by cutting back on the amount of processed foods used. Use more fresh ingredients instead. For example, instead of store-bought pasta sauce, make fresh sauce from scratch. Other foods to avoid include:

o   Frozen pizza

o   Frozen dinners

o   Packaged pasta, grain mixes, and flavored rice

o   Snack foods like salted pretzels, chips and crackers

o   Canned vegetables, soups, and broths

o   Condiments like barbeque sauce, soy sauce, and ketchup

•   Choose less-sodium style of food preparation. For example, use fresh skinless, lean meat and poultry instead of processed, smoked or canned ones. These processes use lots of salt.

•   Learn to cook at home. This allows for greater control over how much salt goes into food. Foods from restaurants and fast-food establishments typically contain lots of salt. It is also difficult to obtain information on the exact amount of salt added to food, making it difficult to make adjustments on daily sodium intake.

•   Salt is not the only thing that gives flavor to food. Learn other flavors from the various herbs and spices available. Fruits like limes and lemons give a nice refreshing flavor to foods without having to use additional salt.

CHAPTER 10

DASH Diet Seven-Day Meal Plan

This is a seven-day meal plan that will help you see how DASH eating looks like. You can use this diet plan to start your journey to lower BP, weight loss and better health.

Do note that this is based on a 2, 000 calorie per day diet. Also, take note that the daily calorie intake should not always be exactly 2, 000 calories. There are days when calorie intake may exceed the recommendation a bit. This can be balanced out by days where calorie intake is less than 2, 000 calories.

1ˢᵗ Day

For Breakfast

- 1 store-bought whole wheat bagel, spread with 2 tablespoons of no-added-salt peanut butter

- 1 medium-sized orange

- Decaffeinated coffee

- 1 cup fat-free milk

For Lunch

- 12 pieces reduced-sodium wheat crackers

- Spinach salad:

- o   4 cups fresh spinach leaves

- o   1/2 cup canned mandarin orange sections

- o   1 sliced pear

- o   2 tablespoons red wine vinaigrette

- o   1/3 cup slivered almonds

- 1 cup fat-free milk

For Dinner

- 3 ounces herb-crusted baked cod

- 1/2 cup brown rice pilaf with vegetables

- 1/2 cup steamed fresh green beans

- 1 small sourdough roll

- 1 cup fresh berries and some chopped mint

- 2 teaspoons olive oil

- 1 glass of herbal iced tea

For snacks (eaten anytime of the day)

- 4 vanilla wafers

- 1 cup low-calorie, fat-free yogurt

Nutritional Analysis

- Calories: 2,015

- Total fat: 70 g

- Monounsaturated fat: 25 g

- Saturated fat: 10 g

- Cholesterol: 70 mg

- Trans fat: 0 g

- Total carbohydrate: 267 g

- Sugars: 109 g

- Dietary fiber: 39 g

- Protein: 90 g

- Potassium: 3,274 mg

- Sodium: 1,607 mg

- Calcium: 1,298 mg

- Magnesium: 394 mg

DASH servings

- Vegetables: 5

- Grains & grain products: 7

- Fruits: 4

- Meats, fish & poultry: 3

- Dairy foods (fat-free or low-fat): 3

- Fats and oils: 3

- Nuts, dry beans & seeds: 2

- Sweets: 1

2ⁿᵈ **Day**

For Breakfast

- 1 bran muffin with 1 teaspoon of trans-fat-free margarine

- 1 cup mixed fresh fruits, example: banana, apple, berries and melons, topped with 1/3 cup toasted walnuts and 1 cup fat-free, vanilla-flavored low-calorie yogurt

- 1 cup fat-free milk

- 1 glass of herbal tea

For Lunch

- Curried chicken wrap:

  - 1 medium whole wheat tortilla

  - 2/3 cup chopped cooked chicken

  - 1/2 cup raw baby carrots

- o   1/2 cup chopped apple

- o   2 tablespoons light mayonnaise

- o   1/2 teaspoon curry powder

- 1 cup fat-free milk

For Dinner

- 1 cup cooked whole wheat spaghetti mixed with 1 cup marinara sauce (do not add any salt)

- 1 whole wheat roll

- 2 cups mixed salad greens drizzled with 1 teaspoon olive oil and tossed with 1 tablespoon Caesar dressing, low-fat

- 1 nectarine

- Sparkling water

For snacks (eaten anytime of the day)

- Trail mix made with:

  - o   1 ounce mini twist pretzels, unsalted varietty

  - o   1/4 cup raisins

  - o   2 tablespoons sunflower seeds

Nutritional Analysis

- Calories: 2,193

- Protein: 95 g

- Total carbohydrate: 324 g

- Sugars: 135 g

- Dietary fiber: 38 mg

- Total fat: 70 g

- Monounsaturated fat: 16 g

- Saturated fat: 11 g

- Cholesterol: 99 mg

- Trans fat: 0 g

- Potassium: 4,219 mg

- Calcium: 1,370 mg

- Sodium: 1,854 mg

- Magnesium: 495 mg

DASH Servings

- Vegetables: 5

- Grains and grain products: 7

- Fruits: 5

- Meats, poultry & fish: 3

- Dairy foods (fat-free or low-fat): 3

- Fats and oils: 3

- Nuts, seeds & dry beans: 2

- Sweets: 0

3rd Day

For Breakfast

- 1 cup cooked old-fashioned oatmeal sprinkled with 1 teaspoon cinnamon

- 1 banana

- 1 slice whole wheat toast with 1 teaspoon trans-fat-free margarine

- 1 cup fat-free milk

For Lunch

- 8 Melba toast crackers

- Tuna salad served over 2 cups romaine lettuce

*for tuna salad

- o 1/2 cup unsalted water-packed tuna, drained

- o 15 grapes

- o 2 tablespoons mayonnaise, fat-free variety

- o 1/4 cup diced celery

- 1 cup fat-free milk

For Dinner

- Beef and vegetable kebab:

  - o 1 cup of cherry tomatoes, mushrooms onions and peppers

  - o 3 ounces of beef

- 1 cup cooked wild rice

- 1 cup pineapple chunks

- 1/3 cup pecans

- Cran-raspberry spritzer:

  - o 4 to 8 ounces of sparkling water

  - o 4 ounces cran-raspberry juice

For snacks (eaten anytime of the day)

- 1 medium peach

- 1 cup light yogurt

Nutritional Analysis

- Calories: 1,868

- Total carbohydrate: 277 g

- Dietary fiber: 29 g

- Sugars: 125 g

- Total fat: 45 g

- Cholesterol: 114 mg

- Monounsaturated fat: 19 g

- Saturated fat: 0 g

- Trans fat: 7 g

- Protein: 103 g

- Potassium: 4,170 mg

- Calcium: 1,083 mg

- Sodium: 1,332 mg

- Magnesium: 423 mg

DASH Servings

- Grains & grain products: 6

- Vegetables: 5

- Fruits: 5

- Dairy foods (low-fat or fat-free): 3

- Meats, poultry and fish: 6

- Nuts, seeds and dry beans: 1

- Fats & oils: 3

- Sweets: 0

4th Day

For Breakfast

- 1 cup no-added-sugar fruit yogurt

- 1 medium peach

- 1 slice whole wheat bread with 1 teaspoon soft margarine

- ½ cup grape juice

For Lunch

- 1 cup carrot sticks

- 1 ham-and-cheese sandwich

- o   2 slices whole wheat bread

- o   2 ounces low-sodium, low-fat ham

- o   1 slice reduced-fat natural cheddar cheese

- o   2 slices tomato

- o   1 large leaf of romaine lettuce

- o   1 tablespoon low-fat mayonnaise

For Dinner

- 1 cup of Spanish rice with chicken

- 1 cup green peas sautéed in 1 teaspoon canola oil

- 1 cup low-fat milk

- 1 cup cantaloupe chunks

For snacks (eaten any time of the day)

- 1 cup low-fat milk

- ¼ cup apricots

- 1 cup apple juice

- 1/3 cup unsalted almonds

Nutritional Analysis

- Calories: 2, 024

- Carbohydrate: 279 g

- Fiber: 35 g

- Total fat: 59 g

- Saturated fat: 12 G

- Cholesterol: 148 mg

- Protein: 110 g

- Sodium: 2, 312 mg

- Magnesium: 538 mg

- Calcium: 1, 417 mg

- Potassium: 4, 575 mg

DASH Servings:

- Grains: 4

- Vegetables: 4 ¾

- Fruits: 7

- Dairy: 3 ½

- Poultry, fish & meats: 5

- Legumes, seeds & nuts: 1

- Fats & oils: 3

5th Day

For Breakfast

- 1 slice of whole wheat bread with 1 teaspoon of soft margarine

- ¾ cup bran flakes cereals with 1 medium-sized banana and 1 cup of low-fat milk

- 1 cup of fresh orange juice

For Lunch

- 2 slices whole wheat bread with 1 tablespoon Dijon mustard

- ¾ cup chicken salad

- ½ cup slices of fresh cucumber

- 1 tablespoon sunflower seeds

- ½ cup tomato wedges

- ½ cup fruit cocktail

- 1 teaspoon low-calorie Italian dressing

For Dinner

- 3 ounces beef eye of round served with 2 tablespoon fat-free beef gravy

- 1 cup sautéed green beans (using ½ teaspoon canola oil

- 1 baked small potato with 1 tablespoon grated reduced-fat cheddar cheese and 1 tablespoon fat-free sour cream topped with 1 tablespoon chopped scallions

- 1 small apple

- 1 small whole wheat roll with 1 teaspoon soft margarine

- 1 cup low fat milk

For snacks

- ¼ cup raisins

- 1/3 cup unsalted almonds

- ½ cup fat-free fruit yogurt (no added sugar)

Nutritional Analysis

- Calories: 2, 062

- Carbohydrate: 284 g

- Fiber: 27 g

- Total fat: 63 g

- Cholesterol: 155 mg

- Saturated fat: 13 g

- Sodium: 2, 101 mg

- Protein: 114 g

- Magnesium: 594 mg

- Calcium: 1, 220 mg

- Potassium: 4, 909 mg

DASH Servings

- Grains: 5

- Vegetables: 5

- Fruits: 6

- Dairy: 2 ½

- Poultry, fish & meats: 6

- Legumes, seeds & nuts: 1 ½

- Fats & oils: 3 ½

6th Day

For Breakfast

- 1 small whole wheat bagel with 1 tablespoon peanut butter

- 1 medium-sized banana

- ½ cup instant oatmeal

- 1 cup low-fat milk

For Lunch

- 1 cup cantaloupe chunks

- 1 chicken sandwich

  - 3 ounces skinless chicken breast

  - 1 slices whole wheat bread

  - 2 slices tomato

  - 1 large leaf of romaine lettuce

  - 1 tablespoon low fat mayonnaise

  - ¾ ounces natural, reduced-fat cheddar cheese

- 1 cup apple juice

For Dinner

- Spinach salad
  - 1 cup spinach leaves
  - ¼ cup grated fresh carrots
  - ¼ cup sliced fresh mushrooms
  - 1 tablespoon vinaigrette dressing
  - ½ cup cooked corn
- 1 cup spaghetti
- 1/2 cup canned pears

For snacks (eaten any time of the day)

- ¼ cup dried apricots
- 1/3 cup unsalted almonds
- 1 cup no-sugar-added, fat-free fruit yogurt

Nutritional Analysis

- Calories: 2, 027
- Total fat: 64 g
- Saturated fat: 13 g

- Cholesterol: 114 mg

- Carbohydrate: 288 g

- Fiber: 34 g

- Protein: 99 g

- Magnesium: 535 mg

- Calcium: 1, 370 mg

- Sodium: 2, 035 mg

- Potassium: 4, 715 mg

DASH Servings

- Grains: 6

- Vegetables: 5 ¼

- Fruits: 7

- Dairy: 3

- Poultry, fish & meats: 3

- Legumes, seeds & nuts: 1 ½

- Fats & oils: 1 ½

7th Day

For Breakfast

- 2 cups puffed wheat cereal with 1 cup low-fat milk and 1 small apple

- 1 small bagel with 1 teaspoon soft margarine

- 1 glass fresh orange juice

For Lunch

- 1 cup potato salad

- Barbecue beef sandwich

  - 1 hamburger bun

  - 1 tablespoon barbecue sauce

  - 2 ounces beef (eye of round)

  - 2 slices reduced-fat natural cheddar chees

  - 2 slices tomato

  - 1 large leaf of romaine lettuce

- 1 medium-sized orange

For Dinner

- 3 ounces cod served with 1 teaspoon lemon juice over ½ cup brown rice

- 1 cup spinach sautéed with 1 teaspoon of canola oil topped with 1 tablespoon slivered almonds

- 1 small cornbread muffin with 1 teaspoon soft margarine

For snacks

- 2 large rectangles graham crackers with 1 tablespoon peanut butter

- 1 tablespoon unsalted sunflower seeds

- 1 cup no-added-sugar, fat-free fruit yogurt

Nutritional Analysis

- Calories: 1, 997

- Carbohydrate: 289 g

- Fiber: 34 g

- Total fat: 56 g

- Saturated fat: 12 g

- Cholesterol: 140 mg

- Protein: 103 g

- Sodium: 2, 114 mg

- Calcium: 1, 537 mg

- Potassium: 4, 676 mg

- Magnesium: 630 mg

DASH Servings

- Grains: 7

- Vegetables: 4 ¾

- Fruits: 4

- Dairy: 3

- Poultry, fish & meats: 5

- Legumes, seeds & nuts: 1 ¼

- Fats & oils: 3

CHAPTER 11

DASH Diet 30 MINUTE Recipes

Raspberry Muffins

Makes 12 servings

Ingredients

- 1/2 cup rolled oats

- 1/2 cup cornmeal

- 3/4 cup all-purpose flour

- 1/4 cup wheat bran

- 1 cup 1% low-fat milk or soya milk (plain soy milk)

- 1/4 teaspoon salt

- 1 tablespoon baking powder

- 1/2 cup dark honey

- 2 teaspoons grated lime zest

- 1 egg, beaten lightly

- 3 1/2 tablespoons canola oil

- 2/3 cup raspberries, fresh or frozen

To make

1. Prepare oven to 400°F.

2. Place liners in a 12-cup muffin pan.

3. Put milk and oats in a small saucepan and cook over medium low heat until creamy and oats are tender. You may cook in a microwave, set on high for about 3 minutes.

4. Set aside cooked oats.

5. Mix cornmeal, flour, salt, bran and baking powder in a separate bowl. Sift or simply whisk together in a bowl.

6. Add lime zest, egg, cooked oats, canola oil and honey.

7. Mix until everything is just moistened but still a bit lumpy.

8. Add raspberries and gently fold into the mixture.

9. Fill each muffin cup 2/3 full.

10. Bake in the preheated oven for 16-18 minutes. The tops should be golden brown and an inserted toothpick (or cake tester) at the center should come out clean.

11. Remove from oven and transfer muffins on a wire rack. Cool before serving.

Nutrition profile:

(per muffin)

- Total carbohydrates: 27 g

- Sodium: 126 mg

- Dietary fiber: 2 g

- Total fat: 5 g

- Saturated fat: 0.5 g

- Monounsaturated fat: 3 g

- Cholesterol: 16 mg

- Trans fat: <0.5

- Protein: 3 g

- Added sugars: 11 g

- Calories: 165

DASH Diet servings

Each muffin is equivalent to 1 serving of:

- Grains, grain products

- Fruits

- Fats & oils

Buckwheat Pancakes with Strawberries

Makes 6 servings

Ingredients

- 2 egg whites

- 1/2 cup fat-free milk

- 1 tablespoon canola oil

- 1/2 cup buckwheat flour

- 1/2 cup plain all-purpose flour

- 1 tablespoon baking powder

- 1/2 cup sparkling water

- 1 tablespoon sugar

- 3 cups sliced fresh strawberries

To make

1. Whisk milk, canola oil and egg whites in a bowl.

2. Combine sugar, flours and baking powder in a separate bowl.

3.   Pour in egg mixture into the dry mixture.

4.   Add sparkling water and mix until everything is slightly moistened.

5.   Heat a griddle or frying pan over medium heat.

6.   Once hot enough, pour half of the pancake batter into the griddle/pan.

7.   Cook until the surface forms bubbles and edges become slightly browned.

8.   Flip the pancake and cook until well browned.

9.   Transfer pancake into a plate.

10.   Cook the remaining batter.

11.   Top pancakes with sliced strawberries. Eat while warm.

Nutritional profile:

(per pancake)

- Total carbohydrates: 24 g

- Sodium: 150 mg

- Dietary fiber: 3 g

- Total fat: 3 g

- Saturated fat: trace amounts

- Monounsaturated fat: 2 g

- Cholesterol: trace amounts

- Protein: 5 g

- Calories: 143

DASH Diet servings

Each pancake is equivalent to:

- 1 serving of grains, grain products food group

- 1 serving of fats & oils food group

- ½ fruit serving

Cranberry Walnut Oatmeal

Makes 1 serving

Ingredients

- 1/3 cup soy milk or skim milk

- 1/4 cup cranberry sauce, unsweetened

- 1/4 cup old-fashioned rolled oats

- 1/4 cup plain low-fat Greek yogurt

- 1/4 cup diced cranberries

- 1 1/2 teaspoons chopped walnuts

- 1/4 teaspoon cinnamon

To make

1. Put all ingredients in a large mason jar.

2. Close the lid tightly and shake the jar to combine everything well.

3. Chill in the refrigerator overnight.

Nutritional profile

(Per 1 cup serving)

- Total carbohydrates: 30 g

- Sodium: 89 mg

- Dietary fiber: 6 g

- Total fats: 4 g

- Saturated fat: 0 g

- Monounsaturated fat: 1 g

- Trans fat: 0 g

- Cholesterol: 4 mg

- Protein: 11 g

- Added sugars: 17 g

- Calories: 193

DASH Diet servings

Each 1 cup serving provides:

- ½ serving of grains & grain products food group

- ½ fruit serving

- ½ serving of fat-free or low-fat dairy food group

Sun-Dried Tomato Basil Pizza

Makes 4 servings

Ingredients

- 1 12-inch pizza crust

- 1/2 cup fat-free ricotta cheese

- 4 garlic cloves, minced

- 1/2 cup sun-dried dry-packed tomatoes

- 1 teaspoon dried thyme

- 2 teaspoons dried basil

To make

1. Soaked tomatoes in water to rehydrate for a few minutes. Once less wrinkly and a bit plump, drain. Coarsely chop and set aside.

2. Prepare oven to 425°F.

3. Prepare a round 12-inch baking pan, coated lightly with cooking spray.

4. Roll out the pizza dough.

5. Press dough into the prepared pan.

6. Sprinkle cheese, garlic and tomatoes over the dough.

7. Top with thyme and basil.

8. Bake in the preheated oven until the crust turns brown. Toppings should also be evenly hot. Bake for about 20 minutes.

9. Slice pizza into 8 equal triangles. Serve hot.

Nutritional profile

1 serving= 2 slices

- Total fats: 5 g

- Sodium: 283 mg

- Total carbohydrate: 33 g

- Dietary fiber: 4 g

- Monounsaturated fat: trace amounts

- Saturated fat: 1 g

- Cholesterol: 7 mg

- Trans fat: 0 g

- Added sugars: 0 g

- Protein: 9 g

- Calories: 216

DASH Diet servings

For a 2-slice serving:

- 2 servings of grains & grain products food group

- 1 vegetable serving

- 1 serving of fats & oils

Chicken in White Wine and Mushroom Sauce

Makes 4 servings

Ingredients

- 4 4-ounce skinless, boneless chicken breast halves

- 2 tablespoons olive oil

- 1/4 pound mushrooms, thinly sliced

- 4 shallots, sliced thinly

- 1 tablespoon plain all-purpose flour

- 1/2 cup low-sodium chicken stock

- 1/4 cup white wine

- 2 tablespoons chopped parsley

- 1 tablespoon fresh rosemary

To make

1. Arrange chicken breasts on parchment paper. Cover with another piece of parchment paper and pound it flat with a mallet.

2. Cover flattened chicken with cling wrap and chill until firm.

3.   Heat 1 tablespoon olive oil in a small pan over medium heat.

4.   Put shallots into the hot pan and sauté until translucent.

5.   Add mushrooms. Cook for 2 more minutes.

6.   While sautéing, mix flour and wine in a small bowl. Whisk until no lumps are present.

7.   Slowly pour flour mixture into the pan with mushrooms and shallots.

8.   Stir continuously until sauce thickens.

9.   Remove pan from heat.

10.   Place rosemary into the pan while still hot then set aside.

11.   Place a large skillet over medium heat.

12.   Heat remaining oil and add chicken.

13.   Sauté until chicken is no longer pink. Internal meat temperature should be 170°F.

14.   Place cooked chicken on a plate.

15.   Pour warm white wine mushroom sauce over chicken.

16.   Serve immediately with a garnish of parsley.

Nutritional profile

(Per serving of 1 half of a chicken breast)

- Total carbohydrate: 5 g

- Sodium: 65 mg

- Dietary fiber: 1 g

- Total fat: 10 g

- Monounsaturated fat: 6 g

- Saturated fat: 2 g

- Trans fat: trace amounts

- Cholesterol: 83 mg

- Protein: 28 g

- Added sugars: 0 g

- Calories: 222

DASH Diet servings

For every chicken breast half:

- 1 vegetable serving

- 4 servings of poultry, fish, meat food group

- 1 serving of fats & oils food group

DASH Delicious Chicken Burritos

Makes 4 servings

Ingredients

- 1 teaspoon olive oil

- 1 jalapeno pepper, sliced

- 1 red bell pepper, sliced

- 1 yellow onion, sliced

- 2 ribs celery, sliced

- 2 cups grape tomatoes

- 2 tablespoons fresh oregano

- 2 tablespoons cumin seeds

- 2 cloves garlic, chopped

- 4 whole-wheat tortillas

- 8 ounces precooked chicken breast meat

- 2 cups shredded green cabbage

- 1/2 cup shredded sharp cheddar cheese

To make

1.	Heat oil in a large skillet placed over medium high heat.

2.	Add celery, pepper, cumin and onions. Sauté for 10-15 minutes until vegetables are lightly brown.

3.	Add garlic, oregano and tomatoes.

4.	Sauté until tomatoes stat to blister then break open.

5.	Remove pan from heat and pour everything in a blender. Puree until the desired consistency is achieved. Transfer to a bowl and set aside.

6.	Shred chicken meat. Divide among the tortillas.

7.	Put cheese on top of the chicken.

8.	Top with cabbage.

9.	Spoon over some of the pureed sauce.

10.	Carefully roll the tortilla and serve immediately.

Nutritional profile

(Per 1 burrito serving)

- Total carbohydrate: 38 g

- Sodium: 486 mg

- Dietary fiber: 12 g

- Total fat: 10 g

- Monounsaturated fat: 3 g

- Saturated fat: 4 g

- Trans fat: 0 g

- Cholesterol: 63 mg

- Protein: 29 g

- Added sugars: 0 g

- Calories: 350

DASH Diet servings

For each burrito:

- 1.5 servings of grains & grain products food group

- 2 servings of vegetables

- 2 servings of poultry, fish & meats food group

- 0.5 servings of dairy food group (fat-free or low fat)

Roasted Salmon with Chives and Tarragon

Makes 2 servings

Ingredients

- 2 5-ounce pieces salmon, skin on

- 2 teaspoons extra-virgin olive oil

- 1 tablespoon fresh tarragon leaves

- 1 tablespoon chopped chives

To make

1. Prepare a 425°F oven.

2. Prepare a baking sheet lined with foil.

3. Rub olive oil all over the salmon pieces.

4. Place salmon with skin-side down on the prepared baking sheet.

5. Bake for 10-12 minutes until salmon flakes readily when pierced with a fork.

6. Remove the skin from the salmon with a metal spatula.

7.   Sprinkle the herbs over the fish and serve immediately.

Nutritional profile

(Per serving of 1 fillet)

- Total carbohydrate: trace amounts

- Dietary fiber: trace amounts

- Sodium: 62 mg

- Total fat: 14 g

- Monounsaturated fat: 6 g

- Saturated fat: 2 g

- Trans fat: 0 g

- Cholesterol: 78 mg

- Protein: 28 g

- Added sugars: trace amounts

- Calories: 244

To make

For each fillet:

- 1 serving of fats & oils food group

- 4 servings of poultry, fish & meats food group

Broiled Scallops with Sweet Lime Sauce

Makes 4 servings

Ingredients

- 1 pound bay or sea scallops, rinsed and patted dry

- 4 tablespoons honey

- 1 tablespoon olive or canola oil

- 2 tablespoons lime juice

- 2 teaspoons grated lime peel

- 1 lime, cut into 4 wedges

To make

1. Heat broiler and place rack 4 inches above the source of heat.

2. Line a cookie sheet or broiler pan with aluminum foil. Spray with oil.

3. Whisk lime juice, oil and honey in a large bowl.

4. Gently toss in the scallops. Coat well.

5.   Place scallops in a single layer on the prepared pan or cookie sheet.

6.   Broil scallops until opaque. Turn scallops over and cook the other side.

7.   Place scallops in the serving plates.

8.   Spoon juices from the pan over the scallops.

9.   Garnish with lime wedge and lime peel.

10.   Serve.

Nutritional profile

(Per 4-ounce serving)

- Total carbohydrate: 23 g

- Sodium: 445 mg

- Dietary fiber: 1 mg

- Total fat: 4 g

- Monounsaturated fat: 2.5 g

- Saturated fat: 1 g

- Trans fat: trace amounts

- Cholesterol: 27 mg

- Protein: 14 g

- Added sugars: 17 g

- Calories: 185

DASH Diet servings

- 2 servings of poultry, fish & meats food group

- 1 serving of sweets food group

Triple Berry Spinach Salad

Makes 4 servings

Ingredients

- 4 cups torn fresh spinach, packed

- 1 cup, blueberries, fresh or frozen

- 1 cup sliced fresh strawberries

- 1/4 cup chopped toasted pecans

- 1 small sweet onion, chopped

Salad dressing:

- 2 tablespoons balsamic vinegar

- 2 tablespoons white wine or cider vinegar

- 2 teaspoons Dijon mustard

- 2 tablespoons honey

- 1/8 teaspoon pepper

- 1 teaspoon curry powder

To make

1. Toss onions, pecans, blueberries, strawberries and spinach in a large bowl.

2. Mix all ingredients for the dressing in a small jar. Close the lid tightly and shake well.

3. Pour dressing over the salad and toss. Coat everything well.

4. Serve.

Nutritional profile

(Per 1 ½ cup serving)

- Total carbohydrate: 25 g

- Dietary fiber: 4 g

- Sodium: 198 mg

- Saturated fat: 0.5 g

- Total fat: 5 g

- Trans fat: 0 g

- Cholesterol: 0 mg

- Protein: 4 g

- Monounsaturated fat: 3 g

- Calories: 158

- Added sugars: 19 g

DASH Diet servings

Each 1 ½ cup serving:

- ½ serving of sweets food group

- 1 serving of vegetables

- ½ serving of seeds, dry beans & nuts food group

- 1 serving of fruit

Simple Mango Salad

Makes 4 servings

Ingredients

- 2 cups diced mangoes

- 1/3 cup minced red onion

- 2 tablespoons minced cilantro

- 1/3 cup minced red Fresno peppers

- 1 tablespoon olive oil

- Juice and zest of 1 lime

To make

1. Toss all ingredients in a bowl.

2. Serve immediately or chill before serving.

Nutritional profile

(Per 2/3 cup serving)

- Total carbohydrate: 15 g

- Sodium: 2 mg

- Dietary fiber: 2 g

- Total fat: 4 g

- Monounsaturated fat: 2.5 g

- Saturated fat: 0.5 g

- Trans fat: 0 g

- Cholesterol: 0 mg

- Protein: 1 g

- Added sugars: 0 g

- Calories: 100

DASH Diet serving

- 1 fruit serving

- 1 serving of fats & oils food group

Cherry Tomato, Basil and Pear Salad

Makes 6 servings

Ingredients

- 1 1/2 cups yellow pear tomatoes, sliced in half

- 1 1/2 cups red cherry tomatoes, sliced in half

- 1 1/2 cups orange cherry tomatoes, sliced in half

- 4 large fresh basil leaves, sliced into slender ribbons

For the vinaigrette

- 2 tablespoons red wine or sherry vinegar

- 1 tablespoon extra-virgin olive oil

- 1 tablespoon minced shallot

- 1/8 teaspoon fresh ground black pepper

- 1/4 teaspoon salt

To make

1. Mix all the ingredients for the vinaigrette in a small bowl. Set aside for 15 minutes to allow flavors to blend well.

2. Whisk in pepper, salt and olive oil to the dressing just before serving.

3. Toss tomatoes and pear in a large bowl.

4. Add dressing and basil.

5. Toss gently to coat everything well.

6. Serve immediately.

Nutritional profile

(Per ¾ cup serving)

- Total carbohydrate: 4 g

- Sodium: 125 mg

- Dietary fiber: 1 g

- Total fat: 3 g

- Monounsaturated fat: 2 g

- Saturated fat: 0 g

- Trans fat: 0 g

- Cholesterol: 0 mg

- Protein: 1 g

- Added sugars: 0 g

- Calories: 47

DASH Diet servings

- ½ serving of fats & oils food group

- 1 serving of vegetables

Tomato Basil Bruschetta

Makes 6 servings

Ingredients

- 1/2 whole-grain baguette, sliced into 6 diagonal slices, each slice 1/2-inch thick

- 1 tablespoon chopped parsley

- 2 tablespoons chopped basil

- 2 cloves garlic, minced

- 1/2 cup diced fennel

- 3 tomatoes, diced

- 2 teaspoons balsamic vinegar

- 1 teaspoon olive oil

- 1 teaspoon black pepper

To make

1. Heat an oven to 400°F. Toast the baguette slices until slightly browned.

2. Place all the remaining ingredients in a large bowl. Toss to mix well.

3. Spoon the mixture on top of the toasted baguette slices.

4. Serve immediately.

Nutritional profile

(per 1 slice serving)

- Total carbohydrate: 20 g

- Sodium: 123 mg

- Dietary fiber: 4 g

- Total fat: 2 g

- Monounsaturated fat: 1 g

- Saturated fat: less than 0.5 g

- Cholesterol: 0 mg

- Trans fat: 0 g

- Protein: 3 g

- Added sugars: 0 g

- Calories: 110

DASH Diet servings

Each 1-slice serving:

- 1 serving of vegetables

- 1 serving of grains & grain products food group

Fruit Kebabs with Lemony Lime Dip

Makes 2 servings

Ingredients

- 6 ounces sugar-free, low-fat lemon yogurt

- 1 teaspoon lime zest

- 1 teaspoon fresh lime juice

- 4 1/2-inch chunks of pineapple

- 1 kiwi, peeled then quartered

- 4 strawberries

- 4 red grapes

- 1/2 banana, sliced into 4 1/2-inch chunks

- 4 wooden skewers

To make

1. Whisk lime zest, lime juice and yogurt in a small bowl. Cover and chill.

2. Arrange each piece of fruit on skewers.

3. Serve fruit skewers with chilled lemon-lime dip.

Nutritional profile

(per serving of 2 kebabs)

- Total carbohydrate: 39 mg

- Sodium: 53 mg

- Dietary fiber: 4 g

- Total fat: 2 g

- Monounsaturated fat: trace amounts

- Saturated fat: 1 g

- Trans fat: 0 g

- Cholesterol: 5 mg

- Protein: 4 g

- Added sugars: 6 g

- Calories: 190

DASH Diet servings

- 2 servings of fruits

- ½ serving of dairy food group (fat-free or low fat)

Homemade Hummus

Makes 14 servings

Ingredients

- 2 16-ounce cans reduced-sodium garbanzos, reserve 1/4 cup liquid, rinsed garbanzos then drain

- 1/4 cup lemon juice

- 1 tablespoon extra-virgin olive oil

- 2 cloves of garlic, minced

- 1/4 teaspoon paprika

- 1/4 teaspoon cracked black pepper

- 3 tablespoons sesame paste or tahini

- 2 tablespoons chopped Italian flat-leaf parsley

To make

1. Puree garbanzos in a food processor or blender.

2. Add parsley, tahini, paprika, pepper, garlic, lemon juice and olive oil.

3. Blend well to get a smooth mixture.

4. Add the reserve garbanzos liquid (from the can), 1 tablespoon at a time. Keep adding until a smooth, thick paste is achieved.

5. Serve immediately.

6.   Hummus can be covered and chilled for later use.

Nutritional profile

(Per ¼ cup serving)

- Total carbohydrate: 10 g

- Sodium: 182 mg

- Dietary fiber: 2.5 g

- Total fat: 3 g

- Monounsaturated fat: 1 g

- Saturated fat: less than 1 g

- Cholesterol: 0 mg

- Trans fat: 0 g

- Protein: 3 g

- Added sugars: 0 g

- Calories: 79

DASH Diet servings

For a ¼ cup serving:

- ½ serving of dry beans, seeds & nuts food group

Artichoke Dip

Makes 8 servings

Ingredients

- 2 cups artichoke hearts

- 4 cups chopped spinach

- 1 tablespoon black pepper

- 1 teaspoon minced thyme

- 1 tablespoon minced parsley

- 2 garlic cloves, minced

- 1 cup white beans, prepared

- 1/2 cup low-fat sour cream

- 2 tablespoons Parmesan cheese

To make

1. Combine all of the ingredients in a large bowl. Mix well.

2. Place in a ceramic or glass baking dish.

3. Bake in a preheated 350°F oven for 30 minutes.

4.   Serve dip warm with vegetables, crackers of whole grain bread.

Nutritional profile

(Per ½ cup serving; not including food that comes with the dip, i.e., vegetables, crackers or bread)

- Total carbohydrate: 14 g

- Sodium: 71 mg

- Dietary fiber: 6 g

- Total fat: 2 g

- Monounsaturated fat: 1 g

- Saturated fat: 1 g

- Trans fat: 0 g

- Cholesterol: 6 mg

- Protein: 5 g

- Added sugars: 0 g

- Calories: 94

DASH Diet servings

For each ½ cup serving of dip alone

- 2 vegetable servings

- ½ serving of dry beans, seeds & nuts food group

Delicious Glaze for Chicken, Fish or Vegetables

Makes 4 servings

Ingredients

- 1 teaspoon lime or lemon juice

- 1 teaspoon grated zest, lime or lemon

- 1/2 cup chicken broth, unsalted

- 1 tablespoon sugar

- 1 tablespoon chopped parsley

- 2 teaspoons cornstarch

To make

1. Place all the ingredients in a microwaveable bowl.

2. Whisk to combine well.

3. Microwave the mixture on high settings for 1-2 minutes until it thickens and becomes clear.

4.   Serve the glaze immediately over vegetables, fish or chicken.

Nutritional profile

(Per 2 tablespoon of glaze; not including chicken, vegetable or fish served with the glaze)

- Total carbohydrate: 5 g

- Sodium: 10 mg

- Dietary fiber: trace amounts

- Total fat: trace amounts

- Monounsaturated fat: trace amounts

- Saturated fat: 0 g

- Trans fat: 0 g

- Cholesterol: 0 mg

- Protein: 1 g

- Added sugars: 3 g

- Total sugars: 2 g

- Calories: 24

Peach Honey Spread

Makes 4 servings

Ingredients

- 1 15-ounce can unsweetened peach halves, drained

- 1/2 teaspoon cinnamon

- 2 tablespoons honey

To make

1. Mix all the above ingredients in a large mixing bowl.

2. Mash with a fork to create a chunky applesauce-like consistency.

3. Serve immediately or cover and chill for a few hours.

Nutritional profile

(Per ½ cup serving)

- Total carbohydrate: 14 g

- Sodium: 3 mg

- Dietary fiber: 1 g

- Total fat: 0 g

- Monounsaturated fat: 0 g

- Saturated fat: 0 g

- Cholesterol: 0 mg

- Added sugars: 8 g

- Total sugars: 13 g

- Protein: 0.5 g

- Calories: 58

- Protein: 0.5 g

DASH Diet servings

For each ½ cup serving:

- 1 fruit serving

Conclusion

Thank you for reading this book.

I hope you were able to learn a lot about DASH and what it can do for you. Moreover, I hope this book was able to teach you all you need to know about how to live a DASH life.

Take the tips and recommendations in this book to start your journey to a healthier BP and better health. Start with the meal plans and the recipes given in this book. In a matter of days, you will surely be seeing good results. Keep up the efforts and you will soon enjoy the many benefits of DASH.

Lastly, if you enjoyed reading the book, could you please take time to share your views with us by posting a review on Amazon? Having a positive review from you helps the book stay on top of the ranks, so we can continue to reach those who can benefit from the information shared within the book. It'd be highly appreciated!

Thank you once again and good luck on your journey towards better health and a more fulfilling life.

CPSIA information can be obtained
at www.ICGtesting.com
Printed in the USA
LVHW020534120620
657887LV00024B/895